The Guide to
Occupational
Therapy
Practice

SECOND EDITION

Penelope A. Moyers, EdD, OTR/L, FAOTA, and
Lucinda M. Dale, EdD, OTR, CHT

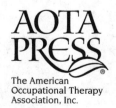

AOTA
PRESS

The American
Occupational Therapy
Association, Inc.

Vision Statement
AOTA advances occupational therapy as the pre-eminent profession in promoting the health, productivity, and quality of life of individuals and society through the therapeutic application of occupation.

Mission Statement
The American Occupational Therapy Association advances the quality, availability, use, and support of occupational therapy through standard-setting, advocacy, education, and research on behalf of its members and the public.

AOTA Staff
Frederick P. Somers, *Executive Director*
Christopher M. Bluhm, *Chief Operating Officer*
Audrey Rothstein, *Director, Marketing and Communications*

Chris Davis, *Managing Editor, AOTA Press*
Timothy Sniffin, *Production Editor*
Carrie Mercadante, *Editorial Assistant*

Robert A. Sacheli, *Manager, Creative Services*
Sarah E. Ely, *Book Production Coordinator*

Marge Wasson, *Marketing Manager*
Stephanie Heishman, *Marketing Specialist*
John Prudente, *Marketing Specialist*

The American Occupational Therapy Association, Inc.
4720 Montgomery Lane
Bethesda, MD 20814
Phone: 301-652-AOTA (2682)
TDD: 800-377-8555
Fax: 301-652-7711
www.aota.org
To order: 1-877-404-AOTA (2682)

Disclaimers
This publication is designed to provide accurate and authoritative information in regard to the subject matter covered. It is sold or distributed with the understanding that the publisher is not engaged in rendering legal, accounting, or other professional service. If legal advice or other expert assistance is required, the services of a competent professional person should be sought.
　　—From the Declaration of Principles jointly adopted by the American Bar Association
　　　and a Committee of Publishers and Associations

It is the objective of the American Occupational Therapy Association to be a forum for free expression and interchange of ideas. The opinions expressed by the contributors to this work are their own and not necessarily those of the American Occupational Therapy Association.

ISBN 10: 1-56900-208-8

ISBN 13: 978-1-56900-208-7

Library of Congress Control Number: 2007920771

Design by Sarah E. Ely

Printed by Automated Graphics, Inc., White Plains, MD

Citation: Moyers, P. A., & Dale, L.M. (2007). *The guide to occupational therapy practice* (2nd ed.). Bethesda, MD: AOTA Press.

Contents

| Tables, Figures, and Exhibits Used in This Publication

Acknowledgments

The authors recognize and thank everyone who reviewed this document, made comments and suggestions, and identified supporting research. Particular thanks go to Carolyn Baum, PhD, OTR/L, FAOTA; Ellen C. Cohn, ScD, OTR, FAOTA; and the members of the AOTA Commission on Practice. Tara Acton, occupational therapy student at the University of Alabama at Birmingham, assisted with identifying the occupational therapy literature.

1 | Introduction

Approximately 40.5 million people in the United States experience disabilities that limit their everyday function (U.S. Census Bureau, 2004). About 2.8 million children ages 5–15 and 13.5 million adults older than age 65 have some kind of disability that greatly affects family life in terms of the need for caregiving and environmental modification. Of people ages 16–64, 21.5 million are affected in their ability to work. Occupational therapy is a service that creates opportunities for people to achieve and maintain function in their occupations and activities related to home, community, and workplace. *The Guide to Occupational Therapy Practice, 2nd edition,* describes the contribution of occupational therapy in

- Facilitating participation of people of all ages in their chosen occupations and activities;
- Designing contexts, environments, and policies for individuals and communities that recognize and support differences in opportunities for participation;
- Improving access to occupational therapy services;
- Enhancing the quality of health care and social services;
- Fostering consumer satisfaction with health care and social services;
- Making possible the appropriate use of health care and social services;
- Reducing costs of health care and social services;
- Preventing disability and impairment;
- Promoting health and wellness; and
- Facilitating the development of children.

The American Occupational Therapy Association (AOTA) represents approximately 36,000 occupational therapists, occupational therapy assistants, and students of occupational therapy. The organi-

zation provides information to support decision making that contributes to health care and social services systems that are high quality, accessible to all, and affordable. This guide describes the scope of occupational therapy practice and outlines the dynamic, occupation-centered process according to an established body of knowledge and the expertise of occupational therapy practitioners.

Occupational therapy intervention and programs lead to improvements in everyone's ability to participate in life situations, regardless of the challenges resulting from disability, health status, or social condition (World Health Organization [WHO], 2001). Occupational therapists and occupational therapy assistants use the term *occupation* to denote self-directed life activities consisting of valued roles and tasks (AOTA, 2002; Baum & Christiansen, 2005b) and use the term *occupational performance* to indicate a complex process of executing occupations and activities that connect individuals to roles and to the sociocultural environment (Baum & Christiansen, 2005b; Reed & Sanderson, 1999). Promoting an understanding of all aspects of occupational performance is the unique contribution of occupational therapy practitioners to health care and to social services provision.

Audience

Occupational therapy practitioners traditionally join their colleagues in medicine, physical therapy, speech–language pathology, psychology, and nursing in offering a comprehensive rehabilitation approach to individuals, populations, families, and others who face a future that has been altered by injury, disease, or health risks. Community-based occupational therapy practitioners emphasize disease prevention and health promotion by organizing and coordinating intervention teams to include social workers, community members and organizations, educators, industry leaders and business owners, architects, lawyers, and public officials. Regardless of whether practice occurs in a medical setting, school system, or organization- or community-based model, occupational therapy practitioners work with people experiencing limitations in occupational performance and inability to participate in the community. Occupational therapy practitioners work to remove barriers limiting individual potential in the performance of valued occupations and activities. They modify environments and activities to match capacities of individuals, organizations, and populations, thereby decreasing the risks for injury, preventing impairment, and promoting healthy lifestyles and habits across the person's lifespan. As the result of the important contributions that occupational therapy practitioners make to the well-being and quality of life of those receiving services, the following audiences may find this guide helpful in understanding and designing comprehensive services that include occupational therapy:

- Occupational therapists and occupational therapy assistants
- Other health care practitioners and social services providers
- Managers of health care and social services organizations
- Health care regulators
- Third-party payers
- Policy analysts, legislators, and other public officials
- Teachers and school administrators
- Community planners and federal, state, and local agencies
- Case managers
- Business and industry leaders
- Clients of occupational therapy services
- Health care and social services researchers and educators
- Foundations and philanthropic organizations.

This Guide—

- Provides guidance and does not preclude professional judgment;

- Represents an overview of the scope of occupational therapy;

- Includes only general methods of program planning, consulting, evaluation, and intervention;

- Requires supplemental information with regard to specific community or organizational issues and conditions, or occupational performance problems of individuals or populations; and

- Does not represent the specific circumstances of individuals, populations, organizations, and communities served.

Use

This practice guide provides an overview of occupational therapy by defining the program planning, consultation, evaluation, and intervention occurring within the boundaries of acceptable occupational therapy practice and the critical reasoning and decision making of the occupational therapy practitioner.

Some examples follow of how this document may be used by occupational therapy practitioners and interested stakeholders:

- To assist occupational therapy practitioners in communicating about services to external audiences and in reflecting on their own practice to maintain competency and to engage in continuing competence
- To assist business and community organizations, health care practitioners, teachers, program administrators, and lawyers in determining the need for and obtaining occupational therapy services for individuals, organizations, or populations

- To assist third-party payers in determining the medical necessity for occupational therapy intervention
- To assist legislators, third-party payers, and administrators in understanding the skills required for occupational therapists to provide program planning, consulting, evaluation, and intervention
- To assist program developers, administrators, legislators, and third-party payers in understanding the scope of occupational therapy
- To assist program evaluators and policy analysts in determining outcome measures appropriate for analyzing the effectiveness of occupational therapy interventions and programs
- To assist policy and health care benefit analysts in determining service needs of given populations that may be addressed by occupational therapy
- To assist community members in understanding how occupational therapy focuses on the identification of barriers to and implementation of strategies for enabling the successful occupational performance of all who live in a community.

Definition of *Occupational Therapy*

The practice of occupational therapy means the therapeutic use of everyday life activities (i.e., occupations) with individuals or groups for the purpose of facilitating participation in roles and situations in home, school, workplace, community, and other settings. Occupational therapy services are provided for the purpose of promoting health and wellness and are provided to those who have or who are at risk for developing an illness, injury, disease, disorder, condition, impairment, disability, activity limitation, or participation restriction. Occupational therapy addresses the physical, cognitive, psychosocial, sensory, and other aspects of occupational performance in a variety of contexts to support engagement in everyday life activities that affect health, well-being, and quality of life (AOTA, 2004a).

The practice of occupational therapy includes the following components (AOTA, 2004a):

- Methods or strategies selected to direct the process of interventions, such as
  - Establishment, remediation, or restoration of a performance skill or ability that has not yet developed or is impaired;
  - Compensation or modification of activities or environments to enhance occupational performance;
  - Maintenance and enhancement of capabilities without which performance in everyday life activities would decline;
  - Health promotion and wellness to enable or enhance occupational performance in everyday life activities; and
  - Prevention of barriers to occupational performance, including disability prevention.
- Evaluation of factors affecting activities of daily living (ADLs), instrumental activities of daily living (IADLs), education, work, play, leisure, and social participation, including
  - Client factors, including body functions (e.g., neuromuscular, sensory, visual, perceptual, cognitive); body structures (e.g., cardiovascular, digestive, integumentary, genitourinary systems); and spirituality, values, and beliefs;
  - Habits, routines, roles, rituals, and behavior patterns;
  - Cultural, physical, environmental, social, and virtual contexts and activity demands that affect occupational performance; and
  - Performance skills, including motor, cognitive, and communication and interaction skills.
- Interventions and procedures to promote or enhance safety and performance in ADLs, IADLs, education, work, play, leisure, and social participation, including
  - Therapeutic use of occupations, exercises, and activities

– Training in self-care, self-management, home management, and community and work reintegration;

– Development, remediation, or compensation of physical, cognitive, neuromuscular, and sensory functions and behavioral skills;

– Therapeutic use of self, including one's personality, insights, perceptions, and judgments, as part of the therapeutic process;

– Education and training, including family members, caregivers, and relevant others;

– Care coordination, case management, and transition services;

– Consultative services to groups, programs, organizations, or communities;

– Modification of environments (home, work, school, or community) and processes, including the application of ergonomic principles;

– Assessment, design, fabrication, application, fitting, and training in assistive technology, adaptive devices, and orthotic devices and training in the use of prosthetic devices;

– Assessment, recommendation, and training in techniques to enhance functional mobility, including wheelchair management;

– Driver rehabilitation and community mobility;

– Management of feeding, eating, and swallowing to enable eating and feeding performance; and

– Application of physical agent modalities and use of a range of specific therapeutic procedures (e.g., wound care management; techniques to enhance sensory, perceptual, and cognitive processing; manual therapy techniques) to enhance occupational performance skills.

Although this definition of occupational therapy helps support the crafting of state laws and regulations that govern the practice of occupational therapy, it does not supersede existing laws and other regulatory requirements. Occupational therapy practitioners are required to abide by statutes and regulations when providing occupational therapy services. State laws and other regulatory requirements typically include statements about educational requirements to practice occupational therapy; procedures to practice occupational therapy legally within the defined area of jurisdiction; and the definition and scope of occupational therapy practice, supervision, and continuing education requirements.

Education, Certification, and Licensure Requirements

Most states, the District of Columbia, and Puerto Rico require occupational therapists and occupational therapy assistants to be licensed (a few states have certification or registration by a state agency). States have similar licensure requirements, including the basic requirements related to education, fieldwork, and certification examination.

To practice as an occupational therapist, the practitioner trained in the United States

• Must have graduated from an occupational therapy program accredited by ACOTE or a predecessor organization,

• Must have successfully completed a period of supervised fieldwork required by the recognized educational institution where the applicant met the academic requirements of an educational program accredited by ACOTE or a predecessor organization, and

• Must have passed the entry-level examination for occupational therapists administered by NBCOT or predecessor organizations (AOTA, 2005c).

To practice as an occupational therapy assistant, the practitioner trained in the United States

• Must have graduated from an occupational therapy assistant program accredited by ACOTE or predecessor organizations,

• Must have successfully completed a period of supervised fieldwork required by the recognized educational institution where the applicant met the academic requirements of an educational program accredited by ACOTE or predecessor organization, and

- Must have passed the entry-level examination for occupational therapy assistants administered by NBCOT or predecessor organizations (AOTA, 2005c).

AOTA supports licensure of qualified occupational therapists and occupational therapy assistants (AOTA, 2003, Policy 5.3). State regulatory agencies may impose additional requirements to practice as an occupational therapist or as an occupational therapy assistant in the area of jurisdiction (AOTA, 2003). AOTA provides guiding documents that often are reflected in state licensure laws and regulations, including the *Model Occupational Therapy Practice Act* (AOTA, 2004a), the *Occupational Therapy Code of Ethics* (AOTA, 2005a), and *Standards of Continuing Competence* (AOTA, 2005b; see Appendix B).

Outcomes of Occupational Therapy

Occupational therapy practitioners use a variety of occupations and activities to promote and maintain physical, cognitive, and emotional health. Engagement in healthy and meaningful occupations and activities creates a person's identity (Christiansen, 1999) and contributes to the quality of life for individuals, organizations, and populations (Bass-Haugen, Henderson, Larson, & Matuska, 2005). Often people with a disability experience environmental barriers, poorly designed activities, and reduced personal capacity so that they are unable to engage in their life activities. Over time, being deprived of routine and important life activities leads to social isolation, perpetuation of the stigma associated with disability, loss of identity, deterioration of health, and dysfunction (Christiansen & Matuska, 2004; Kielhofner, 2004). Occupational therapy practitioners collaborate with individuals, organizations, and populations to design therapeutic occupations and activities that lead to health, accomplishment, mastery, and a sense of purpose and meaning in life.

The overarching goal of occupational therapy is supporting *health* and *participation* in life through *engagement* in occupation (AOTA, 2002):

- According to WHO (1986), *health* is "the extent to which an individual or group is able, on the one hand, to realize aspirations and satisfy needs, and, on the other hand, to change or cope with the environment" (p. 74).
- *Participation* is "involvement in a life situation" (WHO, 2001, p. 10).
- *Engagement* in occupation refers to the commitment made to performance in occupations or activities as the result of self-choice, motivation, and meaning. It includes the subjective aspects of carrying out occupations and activities that are meaningful and purposeful to the person (AOTA, 2002).

Therefore, occupational therapy services achieve outcomes that are important to individuals, organizations, and populations (AOTA, 2002), such as

- Occupational performance, or the ability to carry out life activities in organizations or the community;
- Personal satisfaction;
- Role competence;
- Adaptation;
- Health and wellness; and
- Quality of life.

The research listed in Appendix C supports the efficacy and effectiveness of occupational therapy intervention in producing these outcomes.

Terminology

In this guide, the term *practitioner* refers to both occupational therapists and occupational therapy assistants (AOTA, 2002). When referring to tasks performed specifically by one type of practitioner, the term *occupational therapist* or *occupational therapy assistant* is used (Moyers, 1999).

The term *client* is used broadly to refer to a person, group, program, population, organization, or community for whom the occupational therapy practitioner is providing services (AOTA, 2002; Moyers, 1999). The actual term used for the person receiving occupational therapy will vary by practice setting. For example, in a hospital, the person might be referred to as a patient, whereas in a school, he or she might be called a student.

Components of Health Classification Terminology

The domain of occupational therapy practice recognizes WHO's conceptualization of participation and health articulated in the *International Classification of Functioning, Disability, and Health (ICF*; WHO, 2001). Occupational therapy uses the basic constructs of the *ICF*, including environment, participation, activities, and body structures and functions (AOTA, 2002). Occupational therapy practitioners use the *ICF* because it offers a common language familiar to other health professionals worldwide. Its use is not only a way of enhancing communication about services, but also is a way of organizing and understanding the actual and potential strengths and problems in occupational performance of individuals within organizations or populations. This dynamic and complex relationship between functioning and disability is dependent on the client's health and its effect on body structures and body functions, the activities impor-

tant to the client, and environmental and personal factors.

Although the *ICF* classification is a useful tool for occupational therapy practitioners to communicate with other professionals, it is not sufficient as a professional language for occupational therapy (Haglund & Henriksson, 2003). Occupational therapy practitioners necessarily have their own terminology for describing a person's capacity and the demands of occupations and activities to better guide occupational therapy intervention. Table 1.1 provides a comparison of *ICF* terminology and occupational therapy terminology.

Occupational Therapy Terminology

The occupational therapy profession uses *The Occupational Therapy Practice Framework: Domain and Process* (AOTA, 2002) as a general guide to the use of some of the terminology common in the profession, although theories and research continually inform the precise understanding of and inter-

Table 1.1. Classification Terminology

ICF Terminology Functioning (Disability)	ICF Definition	Occupational Therapy Terminology
Body structure and function (impairment)	Body functions: "the physiological functions of body systems (including psychological functions)" (WHO, 2001, p. 10) Body structures: "anatomical parts of the body such as organs, limbs and their components [that support body function]" (WHO, 2001, p. 10)	Body structure and function
Activities and participation (activity limitation and participation restriction)	"Activity is the execution of a task or action by an individual." (WHO, 2001, p. 10). "Participation is involvement in a life situation." (WHO, 2001, p. 10)	Occupational areas Performance skills Performance patterns
Environmental factors (barriers)	"Environmental factors make up the physical, social, and attitudinal environment in which people live and conduct their lives." (WHO, 2001, p. 10)	Context or contexts and environments
Personal factors	"Personal factors are the particular background of a person's life and living and comprise features of the individual that are not part of a health condition or a health state." (WHO, 2001, p. 17)	Context or contexts and environments

Note. ICF = International Classification of Functioning, Disability, and Health (WHO, 2001).

Supporting Health and Participation in Life Through Engagement in Occupation

Performance Skills	Performance Patterns
Motor Skills	Habits
Process Skills	Routines
Communication/Interaction Skills	Rituals
	Roles

Performance in Areas of Occupation

Activities of Daily Living (ADL)*
Instrumental Activities of Daily Living (IADL)
Education
Work
Play
Leisure
Social Participation

Client Factors	Activity Demands	Environment and Context
Body Functions[1]	Objects Used and Their Properties	Cultural
Body Structures[2]	Space Demands	Physical
Spirituality	Social Demands	Social
Values and Beliefs	Sequencing and Timing	Personal
	Required Actions	Temporal
	Required Body Functions	Virtual
	Required Body Structures	
	Other Client Factors	

*Also referred to as basic activities of daily living (BADL) or personal activities of daily living (PADL).
[1]Body functions (e.g., neuromuscular, sensory, visual, perceptual, cognitive, mental).
[2]Body structures (e.g., cardiovascular, digestive, integumentary systems).
Source: Adapted from AOTA (2002), p. 611.

Figure 1.1. Supporting Health and Participation in Life Through Engagement in Occupation

relationships among the concepts. This edition of *The Guide to Occupational Therapy Practice* updates the *Framework* as the result of feedback obtained nationally and internationally from practitioners, educators, researchers, theorists, students, and external stakeholders (Figure 1.1).

The domain of occupational therapy includes the everyday life activities *(occupations)* that people find meaningful and purposeful. Occupational therapy services enable people to engage (participate) in their everyday life activities within their desired roles, contexts, and life situations. The term *occupational performance* involves the ability to carry out life activities. Occupational therapy organizes life activities into the following areas of occupation (AOTA, 2002):

- ADLs (self-care activities such as grooming and dressing)
- IADLs (complex activities with multiple steps needed to care for self and others, such as household management, financial management, and child care)
- Education (activities related to participating as a learner in a learning environment)
- Leisure (nonobligatory, discretionary, and intrinsically rewarding activities)
- Play (spontaneous and organized activities that promote pleasure, amusement, and diversion)
- Social participation (activities expected of individuals interacting with others)
- Work (employment-related and volunteer activities).

The definition of the term *function,* meanwhile, is essential in occupational therapy practice: Occupational therapy uses the word interchangeably with *performance* and *occupational performance* because occupational therapy's domain is function of the person in his or her occupational roles. Occupational therapy practitioners help people address challenges or difficulties that threaten or impair their ability to perform activities and tasks that are basic to the fulfillment of their roles as worker, parent, spouse or partner, sibling, and friend to self or others.

Since 1917, occupational therapy has focused its services to enhance the function of individuals with, or threatened with, disability. Its practitioners have focused their efforts on function by using interventions to improve the performance of persons who lack the ability to perform an action or activity considered necessary for their everyday lives. Through a joint effort of the person and the clinician, the person's problems, strengths, and assets are identified, followed by therapeutic interventions, educational strategies, access to resources, and environmental adaptations [compensations or modifications] so the person can accomplish his or her goals. The unique contribution of occupational therapy is that the practitioner creates the opportunity for individuals to gain the skill and confidence to accomplish activities and tasks that are meaningful and productive, and in doing so, increases their occupational performance, thus their function. (AOTA, 1995, pp. 1019–1020)

To understand occupational performance, occupational therapy practitioners consider the following factors:

- Repertoire of occupations and activities in which the client engages
- Performance skills and patterns the client uses
- Environmental and personal contexts influencing participation
- Features and demands of the occupation and activity
- Client factors, such as body functions and structures along with spirituality, values, and beliefs.

Definitions in Occupational Therapy

- *Areas of occupation* include ADLs, IADLs, play, leisure, work, education, and social participation. (Activities and participation level of *ICF*)

- *Performance skills* are the features of action, which includes motor, cognitive, and communication and interaction skills. (Activities and participation level of *ICF*)

- *Performance patterns* involve habits, routines, rituals, and roles. (Activities and participation level of *ICF*)

- *Contexts* are the situations or factors that may influence the person's ability to perform an occupation or activity, including temporal, physical, social, cultural, personal, and virtual environments. (Environmental and personal factors of *ICF*)

- *General activity demands* of an occupation include the objects, space, social demands, sequencing or timing, required actions, and required underlying body functions and body structures needed to carry out the activity. (Activities and participation level of *ICF*)

- *Body structures and body functions* are the client factors that make up or provide the ability to do these activities. Strength, control of voluntary movement, and problem solving are examples. (Body structure/body function level of *ICF*)

- *Other client factors* include spirituality, values, and beliefs.

Occupational therapy practitioners use their knowledge and skills to help clients "attain and resume daily life activities that support function and health" throughout the lifespan (AOTA, 2002, p. 610). Participation in activities and occupations that are meaningful involves emotional, psychosocial, cognitive, and physical aspects of performance. This participation provides a means of enhancing health, well-being, and life satisfaction. Occupational therapy services therefore are provided to the following entities:

- Individuals, family, relevant others, and caregivers (such as family members, teachers, employers, and paid caregivers)

- Groups (such as a family, a class of students, or therapy group)
- Organizations (such as business, industry, or agencies)
- Populations within a community.

Person-based intervention provides services to an individual or a small group. The goal is to promote occupational performance and health that lead to participation in the community. It emphasizes how the interaction among client factors, performance skills and patterns, contexts and environments, and activity demands influences performance of the occupations the client needs and wants to do. The intervention focus is on modifying the environment; promoting health; establishing, restoring, and maintaining occupational performance; and preventing further disability and occupational performance problems.

Population-based intervention provides services to a large group as a whole rather than to individuals or small groups. It emphasizes the incidence and prevalence of common health and disabling conditions within a community. The goal is to determine how to use occupation to enhance the health of people in that community. The intervention focus is on health promotion, self-management, and environmental modification. For instance, the practitioner may design programs to address health disparities related to difficulty accessing and engaging in healthy occupations because of homelessness, poverty, discrimination, or availability of services or resources.

Organization-based intervention may take place at the individual or group level and is designed to enable the organization to more efficiently and effectively meet the needs of the clients and organizational stakeholders. It emphasizes how the mission, values, organizational culture and structure, policies and procedures, and built and natural environments support or inhibit the performance of the organization. For example, to better serve a skilled-nursing facility's clients, an occupational therapy practitioner may recommend environmental modifications to the organization's staff. The environmental modification could involve providing important cognitive cues that improve the functioning of all residents (e.g., different colored walls for each hallway so that residents can easily locate their rooms).

Summary

People have many demands they take for granted until a disability makes the performance of activities within an occupational area difficult or impossible and, according to *ICF* terminology, participation in the community is restricted. Likewise, individuals or populations at risk for occupational performance problems benefit from occupational therapy services to prevent impairments in body structures and body functions, activity limitations, and participation restrictions. Occupational therapy practitioners address the goals of the person to enable engagement and participation in a variety of occupations while using activity to promote health.

In addition to helping clients with basic self-care and ADL skills, practitioners help them acquire the performance skills and habits for assuming roles leading to engagement in such IADLs as home maintenance as well as engagement in the many activities associated with work, education, leisure, play, and social participation. When a disability limits function in the areas of occupation, it may be because impairments in body structure or function are interfering with the needed actions, skills, or habits. Those impairments must be addressed to determine the capacity for recovery and the need for modification or compensation. Occupational therapists evaluate the impact of impairments in sensory functions (including pain), neuromusculoskeletal and movement-related functions, mental functions (affective, cognitive, and perceptual), and cardiovascular and respiratory system functions on the performance of occupations. When possible, occupational therapy practitioners provide appropriate interventions to prevent, alleviate, or substantially reduce the effect of those impairments on daily activity and participation in social roles.

The *ICF* focuses on the impact of the environment or context in supporting and sustaining the activity and participation of individuals and populations. Occupational therapy practitioners additionally facilitate occupational performance through environmental modifications and applied technology. For example, practitioners often partner with engineers to ensure performance of activities and work functions.

The domain of occupational therapy presented in Figure 1.1 will enhance understanding of the following examples:

- A person who is injured on the job may have the potential to return to work, which is an occupational area. To achieve the outcome of improved occupational performance involving return to work, the person may need to address specific body structures and body functions, such as strength or muscle power, endurance, mobility, and stability of joints; specific cognitive skills, such as time management or temporal organization; and the physical context, such as structures and objects in his or her environment (AOTA, 1999a). To prevent further or new impairments that may arise from the design of work activities and the work environment, it may be necessary to modify the work activities, objects used on the job, or other contextual factors.

- A child with learning disabilities is required to perform educational activities within a public school setting. Participation in education is an occupational area for the child. To achieve improved occupational performance in education, the child may need to address specific body functions related to movement-related and sensory functions along with motor skills, such as coordinating movements of the fingers and wrist and maintaining sitting posture during handwriting and other learning activities. The handwriting and other learning activities may require modification to accommodate impairments in body function and difficulty in motor and cognitive performance skills. The physical context, such as objects (e.g., the desk and chair) in the environment (AOTA, 1999a), or other features of the context, such as social aspects, may need modification to support improved occupational performance.

- A mother with a history of substance use disorders is having difficulty assuming her parenting role for the family. Engagement in IADLs and social participation are the occupational areas of concern. She may need to address how her substance use habits have interfered with engagement in ADLs and have affected her body functioning, specifically her mental functions of attention and memory; motor skills, such as coordination; and communication and interaction skills needed for raising her children. To prevent relapse, she must establish new routines without substance use; learn how to cope with daily hassles without the use of substances; and participate in healthy activities, especially those that include her children. The social context requires modification so that she interacts with others who have healthy habits and routines instead of spending time with those who drink and use drugs.

2 | Scope of Occupational Therapy

Occupational therapy practitioners are concerned with the engagement of individuals and populations in meaningful and purposeful occupations in the areas of ADLs, IADLs, work, education, social participation, play, and leisure. The term *occupation* is used to capture the breadth and meaning of everyday activity. The philosophical basis of occupational therapy is as follows:

Man [A person] is an active being whose development is influenced by purposeful activity. Using their capacity for intrinsic motivation, human beings are able to influence their physical and mental health and their social and physical environment through purposeful activity. Human life includes a process of continuous adaptation. Adaptation is a change in function that promotes survival and self-actualization. Biological, psychological, and environmental factors may interrupt the adaptation process at any time throughout the life cycle. Dysfunction may occur when adaptation is impaired. Purposeful activity facilitates the adaptive process.

Occupational therapy is based on the belief that purposeful activity [occupation], including its interpersonal and environmental components, may be used to prevent and mediate dysfunction and to elicit maximum adaptation. Activity as used by the occupational therapist includes both an intrinsic and a therapeutic purpose. (AOTA, 1979, p. 785)

In addition, *occupations* are defined as "everyday life activities given value and meaning by individuals and a culture. ... Occupations are central to a person's identity and competence, and they influence how one spends time and makes

decisions" (AOTA, 2002, p. 610). Functioning in one's roles, such as being a parent, employee, or student, depends on successful performance of multiple occupations and activities. Used in this manner, the term *occupation* is more comprehensive than the conventional usage by the public, which refers only to one's vocation (Moyers, 1999). Sometimes occupational therapy practitioners use the terms *occupation* and *activity* interchangeably to describe participation in daily life pursuits, whereas other theorists and researchers in occupational therapy may have distinct meanings for each term. In this guide, the two terms are used together.

Participation restrictions, activity limitations, and impairments—or risks for those problems—may constrain, restrict, or reduce engagement in occupations and activities, thus contributing to a lifestyle of inactivity that may lead to further physical, cognitive, and psychological complications and eventual declines in health.

"Occupational therapy focuses on enabling individuals and groups to participate in everyday occupations that are meaningful to them, provide fulfillment, and engage them in everyday life with others" (Law, 2002b, p. 640). The resources of the individual, organization, or population, when coupled with the skilled intervention of the occupational therapy practitioner, often can effectively resolve occupational performance limitations (Baum & Christiansen, 2005b).

Occupational therapy practitioners are experts in understanding the multidimensional nature of occupations and activities and their effect on the health and wellness of the individual, organization, or population. To fully understand the complexity of occupational performance, occupational therapy practitioners engage in a critical reasoning process involving *general* and *specific activity analyses* and *activity synthesis* (Crepeau, 2003; Kramer & Hinojosa, 2000):

- A general "activity analysis addresses the typical demands of an activity, the range of skills involved in its performance, and the various cultural meanings that might be ascribed to it" (Crepeau, 2003, p. 192). The occupational therapy practitioner uses this knowledge from the general activity analysis to determine the potential of activities and occupations to meet the therapeutic goals of the individual or population.
- The specific activity analysis "takes into account the particular person's interests, goals, abilities, and contexts, as well as the demands of the activity itself" (Crepeau, 2003, p. 193). The details from the specific activity analysis

are necessary to assess the match among the client's capacities and performance skills and patterns with the demands of the activity and of the context.

- When a gap exists between the activity demand and the capacity of the client, the occupational therapy practitioner synthesizes or modifies the activity to create the "just-right challenge" (Kramer & Hinojosa, 2000; Nelson & Jepson-Thomas, 2003).

To illustrate the multifaceted aspects of occupations and activities, consider the everyday activity of writing a paper or report using a computer, an occupation inherent within the student or worker roles. Table 2.1 shows a general and a specific activity analysis typically conducted by the occupational therapy practitioner. In actuality, both types of analyses are much more detailed and require an extensive knowledge base about human and socio-

Table 2.1. Critical Reasoning Process

Critical Reasoning Tool	**General Activity Analysis** (generic design without knowing the person involved)
Purpose	"Activity analysis focuses on the identification of the activity demands and the performance skills" (Crepeau, 2003, p. 192).
Activity Demands	- Objects used and their properties - Space demands - Social demands - Sequence and timing - Required actions, including motor, cognitive, sensory–perceptual, and communication and interaction skills - Required body structures and functions
Context or Environment	N/A
Brief Sample Analysis: Writing a Paper	*Objects:* Computer, desk, chair, informational resources. *Space demands:* Space for person and objects. *Social demands:* Typically performed alone unless the paper is a result of a group school project. *Sequence and timing:* Conducting research, writing first to last page, proofing drafts and rewriting, meeting deadlines. *Required actions:* Motor skills of maintaining posture of trunk and neck, stabilizing arms, moving fingers, coordinating finger movement; cognitive skills in acquiring information and interpreting to confer meaning; organizational abilities to learn and store in memory the information from the research to construct the paper. *Required body structures and functions:* Mental, sensory, neuromusculoskeletal, movement functions.

(Continued)

Table 2.1. Critical Reasoning Process *(Continued)*

Critical Reasoning Tool	Specific Activity Analysis for Male Student Going to High School (current activity design the person uses)
Purpose	"Considers the particular person's goals, abilities, and contexts as well as the demands of the activity itself" (Crepeau, 2003, p. 193).
Activity Demands	• Objects used and their properties • Space demands • Social demands • Sequence and timing • Required actions, including motor, cognitive, sensory–perceptual, and communication and interaction skills • Required body structures and functions • Other client factors, including spirituality, values, and beliefs
Context or Environment	• Cultural • Physical • Social • Personal • Temporal • Virtual
Brief Sample Analysis: Writing a Paper	*Goal:* To get accepted into the state university to study engineering and to pass English with a grade of at least C. *Objects:* 3-year-old laptop; desk is small, and chair is too low for the desk and does not have arms. *Space demands:* Computer barely fits desk. Shares a room with younger brother. Little room between the desk and his bed. *Social demands:* Is an individual project; has interacted with school and public librarians for assistance. *Sequencing and timing:* The teacher has provided sequence for the entire research paper process and has provided a guide for organization of the paper. The student must organize the results of his library research to enhance the flow of the paper. *Required actions:* Has not learned typing, so uses different method than standard hand placement on keyboard. *Required body structures and functions:* Small space places restrictions on neuromusculoskeletal and movement functions. Heavy demand on mental functions (e.g., attention, memory, perceptual functions), particularly on higher level cognitive functions and expression of written language. *Other client factors:* Values education and desires to do well. *Cultural:* Requirements of high school English class, expectations of teacher and parents to do well, friends often do not study. *Physical:* Desk is located in student's bedroom, which is small and cluttered. Lighting in room is poor, placing heavy demand on eye–body structures and visual body functions. *Social:* Writing the paper does not have a social component, but the student is instant messaging with friends at the same time. Student lives with his 3 brothers and parents. His brothers are playing video games in the room while he is working on his paper. *Personal:* Male, junior in high school, and currently having difficulty achieving academic success in English. *Temporal:* Final deadline is the end of the semester. Two weeks remain in the semester. Homework time is before dinner. *Virtual:* Searching the Web for current information on subject for paper, instant messaging friends while writing paper.

cultural systems and the effect of the environment on occupational performance. Note how the specific activity analysis becomes more precise given the circumstances of the high school student who is writing the paper.

The evaluation process is discussed later in this book. Evaluation determines discrepancies between the capacity of the individual, organization, or population and the demands of the activity; it also analyzes the way in which activity design and context or environment either facilitates or inhibits performance. This guide also describes the intervention process, which incorporates activity synthesis as a key strategy for improving occupational performance. Individuals, organizations, or populations whose occupational performance discrepancies are related to impairments, contextual and environmental barriers, and activity design issues benefit from occupational therapy services.

The role of the occupational therapy practitioner is to help the individual, organization, or population improve or maintain abilities to perform despite impairments, activity limitations, or participation restrictions or risk for these problems. As is illustrated in Table 2.1, however, the ability to perform is only one dimension of any occupation or activity. It is not enough that a person has the performance skills and habits needed for participation in occupations or activities. Occupational therapy practitioners, in collaboration with the individual, organization, or population, consider whether occupational performance has the following characteristics (Rogers & Holm, 2003):

- Value, importance, or significance
- Safety, given body structure, body function, and performance skills and habits
- Adequacy, given the difficulty of the occupation and endurance of the client
- Acceptability, according to societal standards and cultural expectations
- Support from the physical (built or natural), social, and cultural environments
- Efficiency, given the amount of time available

- Desirability, given the level of satisfaction generated.

In summary, occupational therapy practitioners view health and human functioning in the context for living (Burke, 2003) and, to that end, emphasize the following factors:
- A holistic view of individuals
- The uniqueness of each person
- The influence of social systems and culture on occupation and occupational performance
- The significance of occupation to health and well-being
- The dynamic relationship among individuals, occupations, and contexts and environments
- The occupational performance of individuals, populations, and organizations.

Situations for Occupational Therapy Services

Age Groups
- *Infants* engage in occupations and activities related to feeding; eating; learning to explore their physical, social, and cultural contexts and environments; and developing capacities for interaction with those environments.
- The occupations of *children* involve school, play, sports, ADLs, and social participation.
- The occupations of *adolescence and young adulthood* focus on preparation for adult occupations (i.e., education) in terms of selecting and planning for careers, developing intimate relationships, engaging in sports or leisure, and learning to independently manage IADLs.
- *Adult* occupations include those associated with work, IADLs (e.g., home management, childrearing), and leisure.
- After retirement from paid work, *older adults* engage in occupations that reflect their interests and values, in addition to ADLs and IADLs. Their occupations and activities must accommodate declines in personal capacities associated with aging and must be particularly adept at promoting healthy aging (Clark, Azen, Carlson, Labree, & Hay, 2001).

Socioeconomic and Cultural Backgrounds

Because of their concern with activity limitations and participation restrictions, occupational therapy practitioners address the realities of the client's perceptions and experiences (Sussenberger, 2003). Practitioners address the following issues resulting from socioeconomic and cultural barriers (Bass-Haugen, Henderson, Larson, & Matuska, 2005; Wilcock, 1998):

- *Occupational deprivation,* or the reduction of activity options
- *Occupational disparities,* or unequal activity opportunity
- *Occupational interruption,* or a break in continuity of occupational performance patterns
- *Occupational imbalance,* or the inability to spend time in activities needed for adequate health, well-being, and life satisfaction.

For example, a single woman with few financial resources works hard to provide for the needs of her three children. Her children may be at risk for occupational deprivation because money is not available to pay for a variety of summer play activities. They also experience occupational disparity, given the activity experiences of classmates from wealthier families. The mother works two jobs and,

as a result, has an occupational imbalance in that she has little time for parenting, leisure, and other IADLs. The family is facing potential occupational interruption because the rent has increased, forcing the family to consider moving to cheaper housing, if available.

Impairments, Activity Limitations, or Participation Restrictions

Occupational therapy practitioners provide services to improve the ability of the individual or population to fulfill role obligations, to improve performance in occupations and activities, and to resolve or compensate for impairments. For example, consider the occupational therapy interventions that target the different levels of disablement for a person with arthritis (Table 2.2).

Because of costs associated with disability and the continuous need for assistance, and because health problems often can be averted, occupational therapy practitioners also provide services that prevent participation restrictions, activity limitations, and impairments from occurring in the first place. For example, for a business organization, occupational therapists evaluate computer and assembly-line workstations to determine the potential for workers to develop cumulative trauma disorders,

Table 2.2. Sample Intervention and Levels of Disablement for a Person With Arthritis

Level of Disablement	Occupational Therapy Intervention	Therapeutic Purpose
Impairments	Design and fabricate splints.	Reduce inflammation of arthritic joints and maintain joint alignment.
	Combine meaningful and purposeful occupations and activities, exercise, and rest.	Increase range of motion, coordination, and strength.
		Prevent declines in body function.
		Build healthy routines and avoid, modify, or replace occupations and activities that exacerbate symptoms.
Activity limitation	Recommend assistive devices and modified activity procedures.	Improve occupational performance in activities of daily living, work, instrumental activities of daily living, social participation, and leisure.
Participation restriction	Consult with the employer to modify the work station and work activities.	Enable fulfillment of the employee role and the provider role for the family.
		Remove physical and social barriers.

such as tendonitis or carpal tunnel syndrome. In a child care environment, an occupational therapist determines whether the appropriate amount and level of stimuli are available for the optimal development of the children. As a population-based intervention, the practitioner works with a city to select and strategically install larger street signage to better accommodate the visual impairments of older adults.

Regardless of the presence of existing activity limitations and impairments, occupational therapy practitioners work with individuals, organizations, and populations to prevent problems from occurring. During evaluation and intervention, they must determine whether the client can perform the occupation or activity safely without risking further damage to already weakened muscles and joints or accidents as a result of cognitive impairments affecting judgment. At the organizational level, occupational therapy practitioners may suggest modifications of work stations that would ordinarily force workers to maintain poor posture. Likewise, occupational therapy practitioners may recommend modifications of curricula for the population of elementary school children to enhance typical development.

Health Promotion

Occupational therapy practitioners participate in health promotion services, which typically involve the development of supports for healthy engagement in occupations and activities as a method of avoiding the unhealthy effects of inactivity (Clark et al., 2001) and inappropriately designed activity. Occupational therapy practitioners educate the public and organizations about balancing work, rest, and leisure and the importance of actively engaging in meaningful occupations.

For example, through a randomized, controlled trial (Clark et al., 1997) and long-term follow-up of the original participants, Clark and colleagues (2001) studied the effects of occupational therapy intervention involving the promotion of healthy occupations. The group of well elderly clients in an independent–living setting who received occupational therapy had greater gains or fewer declines in physical health, physical functioning, social function, vitality, mental health, and life satisfaction compared with those receiving no intervention and those participating only in social activities. Simi-larly, Hay and colleagues (2002) found that preventive occupational therapy services for independent-living adults were cost-effective in terms of health care costs during and after intervention.

Site of Occupational Therapy Services

Occupational therapy services may take place in a variety of settings. The setting depends on the following factors:

- The diagnosis or disabling condition, injury, or occupational performance problem
- The potential risks for developing disabling conditions or occupational performance problems
- The type of community programming, health promotion, or organizational solutions needed
- The level and number of health care and social services needed by the individual or population
- The ability of the family or caregiver and availability of organizations to provide support or supplemental care and supervision (often referred to as *social capital*)
- The contexts or environments needing modification.

Population- and organization-based intervention occurs in settings where multiple persons experience occupational performance problems (e.g., cities, schools, day care centers, homeless shelters, industry). The settings common in occupational therapy are as follows:

- Institutional settings
- Outpatient settings
- Home and community settings.

Exhibit 2.1 lists typical sites of occupational therapy services; however, the list does not imply that occupational therapy is restricted to those sites. Occupational therapy services continue to evolve into alternative settings that may not be included in this description.

Exhibit 2.1. Settings for Occupational Therapy Services

Institutional	Outpatient	Home and Community
• Free-standing rehabilitation hospital or center • Inpatient hospitals • Inpatient mental health • Inpatient rehabilitation • Nursing facilities • Prisons • Research facilities	• Driver's rehabilitation programs • Hospital outpatient • Low vision clinics • Outpatient clinics • Outpatient office • Outpatient rehabilitation • Partial hospitalization • Research facilities	• City parks and recreation departments • Community agencies • Community mental health centers • Day care centers • Departments of Motor Vehicles • Early intervention centers • Group homes • Home • Hospice • Independent and assisted living • Industry and business • Schools and after-school programs • Shelters and drop-in centers • Subsidized housing and halfway houses • Wellness and fitness centers • Work rehabilitation programs

3 | The Occupational Therapy Process

The occupational therapy process is implemented for individuals and small groups as well as for populations, organizations, and communities. Regardless of the recipient of services, the focus remains on occupation and activity and on enabling participation such that the occupational performance of people within varied contexts or environments promotes health and well-being.

Occupational therapists and occupational therapy assistants have different roles throughout the occupational therapy service delivery process. The occupational therapist ultimately is responsible for all aspects of the occupational therapy service delivery process and is accountable for safety and effectiveness. The occupational therapy assistant works under the supervision of and in partnership with the occupational therapist (American Occupational Therapy Association [AOTA], 2005c). As mentioned in Chapter 1, Appendix A provides a description of the education and credentials of each practitioner, and Appendix B presents the *Standards for Continuing Competence* (AOTA, 2005b) for occupational therapy practitioners.

Appendix D delineates the different roles of the occupational therapist and the occupational therapy assistant, and it describes the supervision requirements for occupational therapy assistants (AOTA 2004b). Appendix E presents the *Standards of Practice* (AOTA, 2005c) in chart form not only to describe the standard occupational therapy process but also to illustrate role differences between the occupational therapist and the occupational therapy assistant. State laws can vary regarding the method and frequency of supervision for occupational therapy assistants. State laws and other regulatory requirements should be viewed as minimum criteria to practice occupational therapy. Ethical guidelines always influence occupational therapy practice to ensure safe and effective delivery of services (AOTA, 2005a; see Appendix F).

Occupational Therapy Process for Populations and Organizations

Providing occupational therapy services to an organization, community, or population facilitates the occupational performance of larger groups of people (e.g., residents of an impoverished community who need better access to health-promoting occupations, children with special needs in a school system, workers in a specific industry). Occupational therapy practitioners directly influence organizations and communities by consulting with leaders to change policy or improve processes and environments and contexts affecting occupational performance. They also may work indirectly to assist the organization or community by conducting evaluation and intervention for organizational or community members.

The *population-based process* is client centered in that community members and potential recipients of the program are involved in each step. The focus of analysis is on the characteristics and health behaviors of a population, including incidence and prevalence of disease, chronic conditions, socioeconomic issues, and lifestyle and environmental problems contributing to occupational performance difficulties (Baum, Bass-Haugen, & Christiansen, 2005). This program-planning process includes specific steps (Fazio, 2001; Perinchief, 2003) that incorporate an evidence-based approach in which the best available evidence, combined with input from members of the population, leads to the answers for each of the questions raised in the programming steps (Soukup, 2000). The program-planning process for populations is as follows:

A. Identify, assess, and analyze the occupational performance needs specific to the target population. (What is the internal and external evidence that indicates a population could benefit from occupational therapy programming?)

1. Develop the external profile of the community.
2. Conduct a trends analysis to highlight potential community issues.
3. Develop the internal profile of the community.
4. Select a target population or populations in the community that could benefit from services.
5. Research the specific target population(s) in more depth.
6. Assess the need for occupation-centered programs.

B. Plan and design occupational therapy programs to meet those occupational performance needs. (What are the evidence-supported interventions for inclusion in the programming? How should the program be financed and implemented for the most effective results?)

1. Generate ideas for potential programs.
2. Develop program goals and objectives.
3. Develop the scope of the program based on evidence for best practice.
4. Choose a potential site of service delivery.
5. Develop indicators of service quality.
6. Select evidence-based program outcome and program evaluation measurement instruments and procedures.
7. Determine projected expenses and resources needed.
8. Project revenue and identify potential funding sources.
9. Write and submit grants, proposals, or business plans.

C. Implement the planned occupational therapy programs. (What process evidence will indicate the need for program modification?)

1. Organize and plan implementation processes.
2. Hire and direct staff.
3. Control to ensure that processes are implemented as planned within the budget.
4. Evaluate process to determine efficiency and modify systems as indicated.

D. Evaluate and account for the outcomes of such programs. (What outcome and program evaluation evidence will be observed during program implementation [i.e., what are the formative evaluation data]? What evidence will be observed following implementation of the new programming [i.e., what are the summative evaluation data]? Subsequent to implementation, should the program be continued, modified, replaced, or discontinued?)

1. Collect and analyze formative and summative outcomes and program evaluation data.
2. Design remedial action in response to formative data identifying problems in outcomes.
3. Repeat formative outcome and program evaluation measurement processes to determine whether the problem has been solved.
4. Reinvestigate if problem remains.
5. Periodically monitor formative outcomes and program evaluation data.
6. Use summative outcomes and program evaluation data to determine need for program continuation, modification, replacement, or discontinuation.
7. Seek additional or continued funding as necessary.

The *organization-based process* focuses on the mission, values, organizational culture, policies and procedures, and built and natural environments of the organization and their impact on the way in which people are able to contribute successfully to the organization's productivity. In industry, for example, the occupational therapy practitioner may develop services for managers, supervisors, union leaders, and employees. Interventions for groups and outcomes of group occupational performance become positive influences on the organization as policies and procedures are modified to support changes in worker safety, productivity, and work quality (Dale, 2004). As the organization changes, it may alter ways of doing business with other organizations, such as working with existing suppliers or seeking new suppliers to modify the inventory of office equipment to include furniture that offers ergonomic solutions. Change in organizational performance related to reductions in accidents or injuries, usage of health care benefits, and improvements in efficiency and quality of work may influence which external stakeholders seek to develop business relationships with the organization.

The following process for planning organization-centered interventions is designed not only to improve the occupational performance of its employees but also to have a positive effect on the way in which the organization meets the occupational performance needs of its clients and consumers. The organizational analysis includes the following activities (Baum, et al., 2005):

- Collect information related to the organization's mission and history, values, goals, activities, funding and resources, stakeholders, and clients and consumers.
- Examine the interaction among the organization's customers and consumers, environment and context (e.g., culture, policy, resources), and organizational activities (current or outdated, and capacity for new or revised activity).
- Determine the enablers of and barriers to organizational change.
- Develop a client-centered plan that is based on evidence and research to improve organizational performance.
- Determine the feasibility of the plan through pilot projects.
- Implement the client-centered intervention plan.

- Evaluate the outcome using both formative and summative measures.

Occupational Therapy Process for Individuals and Groups

As with populations and organizations, occupational therapy for individuals and groups is client centered; it involves collaboration with the client or group members throughout each step (Figure 3.1). When working with an individual or a group, occupational therapy includes evaluating, intervening, and targeting outcomes. *Evaluation* consists of developing an occupational profile and analyzing occupational performance; *intervention* consists of developing an intervention plan and implementing and reviewing the intervention; and *outcomes* involve determining whether participation in occupations and activities in various contexts or environments has been achieved. The process also involves an evidence-based approach in which available evidence is reviewed and communicated to the client or group to support decision making

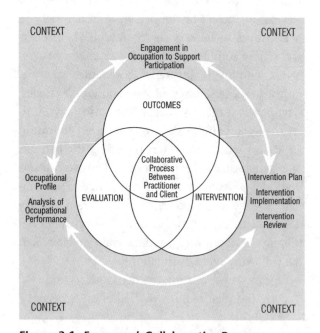

Figure 3.1. *Framework* **Collaborative Process Model.** Illustration of the *Framework* emphasizing client–practitioner interactive relationship and interactive nature of the service delivery process. *Source:* AOTA (2002), p. 614.

throughout the intervention, thus increasing the likelihood of using best practices in selecting methods of evaluation, intervention, and outcome measurement (Ottenbacher, Tickle-Degnen, & Hasselkus, 2002).

Requests for Occupational Therapy Services

AOTA (2004c) states that a referral from a physician or another independent health practitioner (e.g., nurse practitioner, psychologist, or optometrist) is not "required for the provision of occupational therapy services" delivered within a medical model (p. 1034); however, some state laws and other regulatory requirements may require a medical referral. The *Statement of Occupational Therapy Referral* (AOTA, 1994) says that "occupational therapists respond to requests for services, whatever their sources. They may accept and enter cases at their own professional discretion and based on their own level of competency" (p. 1034). A person may independently request occupational therapy services. The occupational therapist may receive requests for services on behalf of the person from a variety of health and social services professionals, teachers and school administrators, family members or caregivers, employers, insurance companies, lawyers, industries or businesses, or state and local agencies. Occupational therapy practitioners also may influence referral patterns through concerted education efforts to potential referrers regarding the benefits of occupational therapy services. Outcome information is provided to the referral source to substantiate the quality of occupational therapy service delivery (Giles, 2003). Requests for occupational therapy services are appropriate when a person is in the following types of situations:

- Unsafe in performing the occupations and activities required in a desired or an expected social role
- At risk for or having activity limitations in the areas of occupation including activities of daily living (ADLs), instrumental activities of daily living (IADLs), work, play, leisure, or social participation

- At risk for or experiencing participation restrictions created by barriers in the context or environment
- At risk for or having impairments in body structure or function
- At risk for or having problems in performance skills or patterns
- In need of healthier interactions among the context and environment and the activity.

Evaluation

Evaluation refers to the entire information-gathering process used to make intervention decisions for people receiving occupational therapy services (AOTA, 2005c; Hinojosa & Kramer, 1998). *Assessment* refers to specific tools, instruments, tests, and interactions that are used during the evaluation process. The results of the evaluation provide a baseline for measuring the effects of the intervention.

In the evaluation process, occupational therapists are concerned with the client's engagement in occupations to support participation in the community or in organizations. Thus, the evaluation process focuses on finding out what the client wants and needs to do and on identifying the factors that act as supports or barriers to performance (AOTA, 2002). The occupational therapist uses theories and evidence to frame the client's occupational performance problems and concerns. The occupational therapy evaluation centers on the *occupational profile* and *analysis of occupational performance* (AOTA, 2002).

Occupational Profile

The *occupational profile* is information that describes the client's occupational history and experiences, patterns of daily living, interests, values, and needs. The profile is designed to gain an understanding of the client's perspective and background (AOTA, 2002). The information should support an individualized approach to the evaluation, intervention planning, and intervention implementation stages of service delivery. The creation of the occupational profile

- Varies depending on the setting and the person,

- Includes information gathered both formally and informally, and
- May be completed in one or multiple sessions. Additional information may be added throughout the occupational therapy process.

The occupational therapist and the occupational therapy assistant (under supervision of the occupational therapist) collect the following information (AOTA, 2002):

- Who is the client (person, caregiver, relevant others, or group)?
- Why is the client seeking services, and what are his or her current concerns relative to engaging in occupations and life activities?
- What areas of occupation are successful, and what areas are causing problems or risks?
- What is the client's occupational history (i.e., life experiences, values, interests, previous patterns of engagement in occupations and in life activities, meanings associated with those activities)?
- What are the client's priorities and desired targeted outcomes?
  - Occupational performance
  - Personal satisfaction
  - Role competence
  - Adaptation
  - Health and wellness
  - Quality of life.

The occupational therapist develops, on the basis of the data, a working hypothesis regarding reasons for occupational performance problems and concerns, identifies the client's strengths and weaknesses related to occupational performance, and determines contextual and environmental barriers and supports. The occupational therapist then preliminarily selects standardized outcome measures.

Analysis of Occupational Performance

The analysis requires an understanding of the complex and dynamic interaction among performance skills and patterns, contexts and environments, general activity demands, and client factors (AOTA, 2002). The purpose of the occupational perform-ance analysis is to gain in-depth understanding of the client's ability to carry out life activities in all areas of occupation, including ADLs, IADLs, education, work, play, leisure, and social participation.

The occupational therapist completes the following steps (AOTA, 2002):

1. Synthesizes information from the occupational profile to focus on specific areas of occupation and their contexts that need to be addressed
2. Uses available evidence and critical reasoning to select the appropriate occupational therapy theories to guide data collection for the evaluation
3. Observes, obtains input from the occupational therapy assistant, and notes effectiveness of the client's performance in desired occupations and activities
4. Selects and uses (or supervises the occupational therapy assistant in using) assessments to measure contexts, activity demands, and client factors that influence performance skills and patterns
5. Interprets the assessment data to identify supports and barriers to performance
6. Develops and refines hypotheses about the client's occupational performance strengths and weaknesses
7. Creates goals, in collaboration with the client, that address the desired targeted outcomes
8. Confirms outcome measures to be used
9. Delineates potential intervention approaches based on best practice and evidence.

Performance in Areas of Occupation

During evaluation, the occupational therapist skill-fully observes the client engaging in selected occupations and activities. To facilitate observation and to focus the evaluation, the therapist selects assessment tools that target only those ADL, IADL, education, social participation, work, play, and leisure activities that are of particular concern to the client and his or her caregivers or relevant others. Those occupations and activities are delineated within the occupational profile. Exhibit 3.1 lists life activities within the areas of occupation.

Exhibit 3.1. Areas of Occupation

ADLs
- Bathing, showering
- Bowel and bladder management
- Dressing
- Eating
- Feeding
- Functional mobility
- Personal device care
- Personal hygiene and grooming
- Sexual activity
- Sleep/rest
- Toilet hygiene

IADLs
- Care of others
- Care of pets
- Child rearing
- Communication device use
- Community mobility
- Financial management
- Health management and maintenance
- Home establishment and management
- Meal preparation and cleanup
- Safety procedures and emergency responses
- Shopping

Education
- Formal educational participation
- Exploration of informal personal educational needs or interests
- Informal personal education

Work
- Employment interests and pursuits
- Employment seeking and acquisition
- Job performance
- Retirement preparation and adjustment
- Volunteer exploration
- Volunteer participation

Play
- Play exploration
- Play participation

Leisure
- Leisure exploration
- Leisure participation

Social Participation
- Community
- Family
- Peer, friend

Source: Adapted from AOTA (2002) pp. 620–621.

Appendix G provides the appropriate procedural terminology for evaluation of occupational performance. Procedural terminology is important to use when working within a medical model because it facilitates effective communication with third-party payers.

Performance Skills
"Evaluation of a performance skill occurs when the performer, the context, and the demands of the activity come together in the performance of the activity" (AOTA, 2002, p. 612). Performance skills are learned functions and abilities and include motor, cognitive, and communication and interaction skills. Examples include actions and interactions with objects (motor skills), such as reaching and gripping; the appropriate use of objects in initiating and sequencing the steps of an activity (thinking, or cognitive skills); and the ability to speak and relate to others as activities are performed (communication and interaction skills). Exhibit 3.2 lists specific performance skills and their definitions. The list is *not* inclusive of all types of performance skills.

Performance Patterns
Performance patterns include roles, habits, routines, and rituals. *Roles* are "recognizable positions in society, each having a defined status and specific expectations for behavior" (Baum & Christiansen, 2005b, p. 253). Typically, a person assumes multiple roles (e.g., mother, sister, spouse, student, worker). *Habits* are "a recurring, largely automatic pattern of time use within the context of daily occupations" (Christiansen & Baum, 2005, p. 546). Habits have the following characteristics:
- They may be *useful,* in that they support performance in daily life (e.g., driving home automatically).
- They may be *impoverished,* in that they have not been established and need practice to improve (e.g., the person must think about each activity regardless of how often it has been completed in the past).
- They may be *dominating,* in that they interfere with daily life or satisfy a compulsive need for

Exhibit 3.2. Occupational Performance Skills

Motor Skills	Cognitive Skills	Communication & Interaction Skills
• *Posture*—the stabilizing and aligning of one's body while moving in relation to activity objects with which one must interact	• *Energy*—sustained cognitive effort over the course of occupational performance while using process skills	• *Physicality*—use of the physical body, such as gestures, when communicating during occupational performance
• *Mobility*—ability to move the entire body or a body part in space as necessary when interacting with activity objects	• *Knowledge*—the ability to seek, discover, learn, and use activity-related information	• *Information exchange*—refers to giving and receiving information during occupational performance
• *Coordination*—the use of more than one body part to interact with activity objects in a manner that supports occupational performance	• *Temporal organization*—the beginning, logical ordering, continuation, and completion of the steps and action sequences of an activity or occupation	• *Relations*—ability to maintain appropriate relationships during occupational performance
• *Strength* and *effort*—skills that require generation of muscle force appropriate for effective interaction with activity objects	• *Organizing space* and *objects*—skills for arranging and assembling activity spaces and objects into ordered wholes	
• *Energy*—sustained effort over the course of occupational performance while using motor skills	• *Adaptation*—the ability to anticipate, correct for, and benefit by learning from the consequences of errors that arise in the course of occupational performance	

Source: Adapted from AOTA (2002), p. 621.

order (e.g., having to check or recheck the door multiple times to make sure it is locked).

- They may be *ineffective* or *inappropriate* for successful occupational performance (e.g., drinking alcohol daily; AOTA, 2002; Holm, Rogers, & Stone, 2003).

Routines are "occupations with established sequences" (Christiansen & Baum, 2005, p. 12), or activities that provide a structure for daily life. *Rituals* share some characteristics with habits and routines but are distinct in that they are routines with meaning. They contribute to a person's identity and thereby reinforce values and beliefs.

While many rituals are cultural and therefore easily recognizable to others within the culture, others are more personal and may be undertaken privately within specific families or by individuals to commemorate special occasions or events or to accomplish other purposes. (Christiansen, 2005, p. 79)

Performance patterns form structure for everyday activities by defining expectations, sequence of steps, and automatic and planned behaviors for occupational performance. During the evaluation, the occupational therapist identifies performance patterns that interfere with occupational performance and those that enhance occupational performance.

Context and Environment

Contexts and environments are conditions external or internal to a person that influence occupational performance. Contexts are varied and include cultural, physical, social, personal, temporal, and virtual. For example, spending time using a home computer, a virtual context, may influence time spent in other leisure activities and IADLs. During the evaluation, the occupational therapist identifies the features of contexts and environments that are relevant to the client and that support or hinder occupational performance. Table 3.1 defines each context.

General Activity Demands

Activity demands are "aspects of an activity, which include the objects, space, social demands,

Table 3.1. Occupational Performance Contexts and Environments

Context or Environment	Definition
Cultural (external features that have been internalized)	Customs, beliefs, activity patterns, behavior standards, and expectations accepted by the society of which the client is a member; includes political aspects, such as laws that affect access to resources and affirm personal rights. Also includes opportunities for education, employment, and economic support.
Physical (external to the person)	Nonhuman aspects of contexts. Includes the accessibility to and performance within environments having natural terrain, plants, animals, buildings, furniture, objects, tools, or devices.
Social (external to the person)	Availability and expectations of significant individuals, such as spouse, friends, and caregivers. Includes larger social groups that are influential in establishing norms, role expectations, and social routines.
Personal (external or internal to the person)	"Features of the individual that are not part of a health condition or health status" (WHO, 2001, p. 17). Personal context includes age, gender, socioeconomic status, and educational status.
Temporal (external or internal to the person)	"Location of occupational performance in time" (Neistadt & Crepeau, 1998, p. 292).
Virtual (external to the person)	Environment in which communication occurs by means of airwaves or computers and an absence of physical contact.

Source: Adapted from AOTA (2002), p. 623.

sequencing or timing, required actions, and required underlying body functions and body structures needed to carry out the activity" (AOTA, 2002, p. 624). These may include the demands of other client factors, such as the person's spirituality, values, and beliefs. For example, use of a conventional computer requires posture to sit in a chair along with the strength, endurance, and coordination to use the keyboard. The occupational therapist evaluates how the activity demands fit with the unique capacity of the client and notes the ways in which the success of occupational performance is influenced by any mismatch between the activity demands and the client's capacity. Once the deficits are identified, strategies for improving performance are determined. Table 3.2 lists activity demands and their definitions (AOTA, 2002, p. 624).

Client Factors

Client factors include body structures and body functions (WHO, 2001), which were discussed previously in the section describing activity demands. Client factors also include the client's spirituality, values,

and beliefs. The occupational therapist considers the categories of client factors listed in Table 3.3.

The occupational therapist selectively evaluates how body structures and functions influence occupational performance both positively and negatively. For example, the arms and hands (body structures) of the client may be unaffected by a spinal cord injury, whereas the legs and feet (body structures) may be impaired. In this same example, the neuromusculoskeletal system (body function) is unaffected for performance of occupations and activities using the arms and hands but is severely limited in performance of occupations and activities using the legs.

It also is important to assess the meaning of occupations and activities to the client as an essential motivator for enhancing the depth of the client's engagement. "To see occupation as the making of lives and worlds is a spiritual perspective" (Peloquin, 2003, p. 124). Understanding the client's spirituality, values, and beliefs helps in the collaborative construction of intervention goals that imagine possibilities and evaluate future choices.

Table 3.2. Activity Demands

Activity Demand	Definition
Objects and their properties	The tools, materials, and equipment used in the process of carrying out the activity
Space demands (relates to physical context)	The physical environment requirements of the activity (e.g., size, arrangement, surface, lighting, temperature, noise, humidity, ventilation)
Social demands (relates to social and cultural contexts)	The social structure and demands that may be required by the activity
Sequence and timing	The process used to carry out the activity (e.g., specific steps, sequence, timing requirements)
Required actions	The usual skills that would be required by any performer to carry out the activity. Motor, cognitive, and communication and interaction skills each should be considered. The performance skills demanded by an activity are correlated with the demands of the other activity aspects (e.g., objects, space)
Required body functions	"The physiological functions of body systems (including psychological functions)" (WHO, 2001, p. 10) that are required to support the actions used to perform the activity
Required body structures	"Anatomical parts of the body such as organs, limbs, and their components [that support body function]" (WHO, 2001, p. 10) required to perform the activity
Other client factors	The demands made on a person's spirituality, values, and beliefs.

Source: Adapted from AOTA (2002), p. 196, Table 5.

Table 3.3. Client Factors

Body Function	Body Structure
Mental functions (affective, cognitive, perceptual)	Structures of the nervous system
Sensory functions and pain	The eye, ear, and related structures
Neuromusculoskeletal and movement-related functions	Structures related to movement
Cardiovascular, hematological, immunological, and respiratory systems	Structures of the cardiovascular, immunological, and respiratory systems
Voice and speech	Structures involved in voice and speech
Digestive, metabolic, and endocrine systems	Structures related to the digestive, metabolic, and endocrine systems
Genitourinary and reproductive systems	Structures related to the genitourinary and reproductive systems
Skin and related structures	Skin and related structures

Source: Adapted from AOTA (2002), pp. 624–626, Table 6.

- *Spirituality* is the "personal quest for understanding answers to ultimate questions about life, meaning, and the sacred."
- *Values* are principles, standards, or qualities con-sidered worthwhile or desirable by the person who holds them (www.apsu.edu/wet/whatis.html).
- *Beliefs* are any cognitive content held as true.

Evaluation Length and Scope

The length and scope of the evaluation are determined by the following factors:

- The likelihood of potential risks leading to limitations in occupations and activities
- The pervasiveness of existing limitations in occupations and activities
- The contextual and environmental factors creating participation restrictions
- The extent of impairments in body structure and function and in other client factors
- The number, severity, and complexity of the disabling disorder, disease, or injury
- The quality of performance skills and patterns
- The demands of the client's activities

- The degree of need for prevention and health promotion.

Occupational therapists use multiple methods to gather data regarding occupational performance. These methods not only involve the client but also include input from family members, relevant others, and caregivers, as appropriate (Exhibit 3.3). Because multiple variables typically influence a person's success in occupational performance and participation, evaluation can be complex. Table 3.4 provides brief examples of how each underlying factor influences occupational performance.

Occupational Performance Problem Statement

Upon completion of the evaluation process, the occupational therapist formulates a performance problem statement to integrate the results from the occupational profile with the results of assessments used to complete the analysis. The occupational performance problem statement succinctly describes the occupational status of the client and identifies the problems amenable to intervention. The statement involves several elements, as shown in Table 3.5.

Exhibit 3.3. Evaluation Methods and Data Obtained

Evaluation Methods	Data Obtained
<ul><li>Self-assessment questionnaires</li><li>Environmental assessments</li><li>Checklists and rankings</li><li>Occupational histories</li><li>Occupational narratives</li><li>Skilled observation of occupational performance</li><li>Performance skill ratings</li><li>Activity simulations</li><li>Standardized tests</li><li>Nonstandardized tests</li></ul>	<ul><li>Premorbid or self-perception of current functioning level in activities of daily living, instrumental activities of daily living, work, education, play, leisure, and social participation</li><li>Interests, meanings, values, and beliefs regarding occupations and activities</li><li>Participation levels in the community</li><li>Health status</li><li>Potential therapeutic occupations and activities</li><li>Abilities and limitations in occupational performance</li><li>Possible goals for future occupational performance</li><li>Contexts and environments that support or interfere with occupational performance</li><li>Performance skill abilities and inabilities</li><li>Inappropriate or appropriate performance patterns</li><li>Body structure and function capacities and impairments</li></ul>

Table 3.4. Evaluation of Influences on Occupational Performance

Underlying Factors of Occupational Performance	As Leading to Problems in Occupational Performance	As Leading to Successful Occupational Performance
Performance skills	Client lacks motor skills for lifting groceries as an aspect of home management.	Ability to use communication and interaction skills enables client to order groceries for home management.
Performance patterns	Grooming habits and routines are inadequate to prepare for school.	Intact dressing habits and routines enable preparation for school.
Context and environment	Noisy, crowded room with people talking loudly makes hearing and following the instructions difficult.	Caregiver creates a safe, cozy space in the living room with pillows, cushions, and blankets for the child to jump, hide, and sleep.
Activity demands	Computer keyboarding to create a document for work demands coordination and motor skills at a higher level than client possesses.	Creating a report for work demands cognitive skills of sequencing and organizing consistent with the person's ability.
Client factors (body function and structure)	Arthritis interferes with performance of activities of daily living (ADLs) because of impaired mobility of hand joints.	Client has mental capacity for problem-solving methods to modify ADL activities.
Client factors (spirituality, values, and beliefs)	Engaging in substance use activities is inconsistent with the person's values related to health.	Family wants to learn how to support the occupational performance of their elderly father because they believe that his participation is crucial to family life.

Intervention

The intervention process includes three distinct steps:

- Intervention plan
- Intervention implementation
- Intervention review.

Intervention Plan

The intervention plan is developed in collaboration with the client, reflects the client's goals and priorities, and is based on the results of the evaluation process, particularly the occupational performance problem statement. Ultimately, the plan describes the specific occupational therapy approaches and types of interventions that will accomplish the client's targeted outcomes (AOTA, 2002, p. 617). In addition to addressing the occupational performance needs of the client, family, relevant others, and caregiver, the setting or circumstances in which the intervention is provided may influence the priority given to problems addressed in the intervention plan. For example, occupational therapy pro-

vided in the school setting is expected to focus on impairments, performance skills and patterns, activity limitations, and participation restrictions that may affect educational performance. Occupational therapists and occupational therapy assistants providing intervention for clients who are unable to work and who are receiving workers' compensation benefits will focus on returning the client to employment.

The occupational therapist develops the intervention plan; the occupational therapy assistant may contribute to its development. The steps are as follows:

1. Establish objective and measurable goals with time frames.
2. Identify the approaches for the occupational therapy intervention on the basis of theory and evidence.
3. Establish the mechanisms for service delivery (e.g., provider of the intervention; type of intervention; frequency, intensity, and duration of service).

Table 3.5. Occupational Performance Problem Statement

Statement Elements	Sample Statement for Person With Right-Hemisphere Stroke
Intervention focus on occupational performance in *prioritized* areas of occupation	Difficulty performing activities of daily living (ADLs); specifically, getting dressed in the morning independently within 15–20 minutes
Intervention focus on *prioritized* activities within the areas of occupation	The dressing activities requiring maximum assistance include obtaining clothing from closet and dresser, dressing and undressing, and fastening and adjusting clothing and shoes.
Occupational performance skills (motor, cognitive, communication, and interaction) as demanded by prioritized activities	Motor-skills impairments leading to activity limitations involve • Problems with trunk control to assume and shift postures during dressing; • Lack of voluntary muscle control of left upper and lower extremities to reach and grip clothing and to transport clothing from dresser or closet to bed; • Lack of coordination during dressing; • Problems in manipulating buttons, zippers, and other fasteners; and • Variability in pacing of activity depending on time of day and other fatigue factors with low endurance decreasing ability to complete task within time frame. Cognitive skill impairments involve • Problems sequencing activity steps in correct order for dressing, • Difficulty searching and locating clothing needed for dressing, • Limitations in maintaining attention to dressing activity because client fatigues easily, and • Termination of dressing activity before completion. Communication and interaction impairments involve • Difficulty articulating speech and • Not making needs clearly known during dressing activity.
Occupational performance patterns (roles, habits, rituals, and routines)	The client lives with his wife and is in the retiree and volunteer roles. Prior to his stroke he had a well-established morning ADL routine and healthy exercise and dietary habits. He and his wife had an early morning ritual of drinking coffee together on the back porch to watch the sun rise. Routines, rituals, and habits have been disrupted by performance skills inabilities and impairments in body function.
Person factors (body structure and function, spirituality, beliefs, and values)	Decreased muscle strength, spasticity and hypotonicity, and lack of voluntary muscle control of arm and leg on the left side of the body. Problems with sensory functions, such as proprioception and temperature sensitivity. Impairments in cognitive and perceptual functions such as memory, higher level cognitive functions, and visuospatial perception. Believes he should have died. Believes his life is meaningless because he no longer can engage in his valued activities. Refuses to go to the Catholic church, as was his habit and belief system, because he reports being angry with God.
Contextual and environmental supports and barriers (cultural, physical, social, personal, temporal, or virtual)	*Personal context support:* The client has a college education. *Social context support:* The client's spouse is able to provide assistance with some of the dressing activity demands. *Physical context barrier:* The lower dresser drawers require the client to bend or stoop, which overly challenges balance. *Temporal context barrier:* The length of time spent on dressing currently limits time and energy available for volunteer, IADLs, and leisure activities. *Virtual context support:* The client has access to a computer and in the past has enjoyed e-mailing family members.

Source: Data from Moyers & Christiansen (2004), p. 74.

In addition, the occupational therapist considers potential discharge needs and plans, selects outcome measures, and makes recommendations or referrals to others as needed.

Content of the Intervention Plan

Exhibit 3.4 identifies and defines the usual content of the occupational therapy evaluation report, which includes the occupational performance problem statement and intervention plan (Sames, 2005).

The initial intervention plan indicates the best estimate of the appropriate frequency, intensity, and duration of intervention. The estimates are updated through reevaluation when evidence begins to accumulate regarding the accuracy of the estimated time frame. Initial estimates of frequency (sessions per week), duration (length of intervention from evaluation through termination of services), and intensity (length of individual sessions) depend on the following factors:

- Degree of impairment, activity limitations, and participation restrictions and potential for change
- Need for prevention and health promotion to support improved health status
- Capacity of the client to develop and maintain performance skills and patterns and the capacity to adapt or compensate for impairments
- Potential to modify barriers in the contexts and environments and in prioritized activities
- Existence of supports in contexts or environments
- Knowledge of intervention outcomes for people with similar conditions or situations
- Information obtained from evidence, research, and outcome studies
- Feasibility of the plan, given the needs of the client, family, relevant others, and caregivers and considering the performance contexts and environments
- Ability of the client, family, relevant others, and caregivers to participate in the occupational therapy program and to access community resources (i.e., social capital)

- Existence of complications or other factors that may slow or accelerate progress.

Goals of Intervention

The goals for intervention are written to define the expected change in occupational performance as a result of the planned intervention. Additionally, goals often include reference to specific and measurable changes in performance skills or patterns and changes in context, activity demands, or body functions that will support occupational performance. The actual style of writing goals may vary by the occupational therapist or by the organization employing the occupational therapist. Regardless of style differences, however, the occupational performance expected as the result of intervention is the well-delineated focus of the goal. Occupational therapy assistants may contribute to the development of the goals.

The purpose of a goal is to indicate changes in baseline performance in occupations or activities that are expected to occur as the result of planned intervention. Improved occupational performance may be reflected in a variety of ways:

- New occupational performance
- Increased frequency of performance in occupations and activities
- Longer periods of sustained performance in occupations and activities
- Reduction in the assistance required for occupational performance
- Greater consistency of occupational performance
- Improved quality of occupational performance
- Decreased time required to complete occupations and activities
- Fewer errors in occupational performance
- Gradation to more complex occupational performance
- Generalization of skills to more occupations and activities
- Elimination of or reduction in aberrant activity behaviors in occupational performance
- Occurrence of pain-free or reduced pain during occupational performance
- Advent of safe occupational performance.

Exhibit 3.4. Content of the Occupational Therapy Evaluation Report and Intervention Plan

Background Information

Typically includes
- Client's name
- Date of referral (if necessary)
- Date of birth or age
- Primary and secondary intervention diagnoses or concerns
- Precautions or contraindications
- Reason for referral or need for evaluation and intervention.

Assessments Performed

Typically includes
- Name of instrument(s) or use of observation
- Purpose of instrument or observation
- Method of scoring or measurement
- Scores and meaning of scores or measurement.

Occupational Performance Problem Statement *(Evaluation Results)*

Occupational Profile
- Prior level of occupational performance
- Concerns, needs, and problems of client, relevant others, and caregivers about occupations and life activity performance
- Priorities for occupational performance.

Occupational Analysis
- Occupational performance problems and strengths in areas of occupation indicated as of concern and a priority
- Specific activity demands creating limitations or supporting abilities.

The rest of the analysis reports only the underlying factors pertinent to the occupational performance problems.

- Performance skill needs, deficits, and strengths
  - Motor skills
  - Cognitive skills
  - Communication and interaction skills
- Performance pattern disruptions and remaining patterns
  - Roles
  - Routines
  - Habits
  - Rituals
- Client factor impairments and capacities
  - Body structure
  - Body function
- Spirituality, values, and beliefs that support and provide meaning for engagement or that interfere with occupational performance
- Contextual and environmental barriers and supports.

Plan *(Prioritization of Occupational Performance Problems)*

- Mutually agreed-on goals
- Recommended intervention approaches, types, and specific intervention methods
- Expected frequency, duration, and intensity
- Location of intervention
- Anticipated discharge environment.

Signature, Credentials, and Date of Report

Source: Data from Sames (2005).

Table 3.6. Sample Goals

Area of Occupational Performance	Goal
Activities of daily living (Dressing)	Within 4 weeks, client will *sequence* dressing activities with *minimal assistance of verbal cues* using *one-handed techniques*. (Cognitive skills and activity modification)
Instrumental activities of daily living (Community mobility)	Within 2 weeks, client will *accurately follow* a bus schedule to independently and *consistently* use the bus system to conduct volunteer duties. (Cognitive skills, development of habit)
Work (Employment pursuit)	Within 2 weeks, client will have the *muscle strength and balance* to use *correct sitting postures* during computer keyboarding. (Body structure and function and motor skills)
Leisure (Leisure participation)	Within 1 month, client will use *interpersonal skills* to engage in leisure activities that allow for *peer relationships* with *those who do not use* substances. (Communication and interaction skills, social context modification)
Play (Play participation)	In 2 weeks, the client will *reach and grasp* a rattle placed 8 inches from the midline by the caregiver and attempt to hand it back. (Activity modification, body structure and function, and motor skills)
Social participation (Family)	In 1 week, client will initiate and *clearly communicate* one *assertive response* to a family member when encountering a confrontation. (Communication and interaction skills)
Education (Formal educational participation)	In 3 weeks, client will use, with *setup*, a *voice-activated computer system* to produce half-page documents for classroom assignment. (Activity modification)

Note. The parenthetical information does not normally occur in practice but is provided here to illustrate concepts. Please note that 4 or 5 opportunities are needed for success and a single performance is not sufficient to meet goals.

Table 3.6 provides sample goals targeting specific areas of occupational performance. The sample goals include various ways of measuring change, such as assistance levels, and delineating the new occupation that the client is expected to perform. The body structures and functions, performance skills and patterns, and activity and contextual or environmental modifications are addressed as appropriate and are highlighted for the reader.

Intervention Approaches

Regardless of the approach used for intervention, the occupational therapy practitioner, in collaboration with the client, focuses on changing the contexts and environments, activity demands, client factors, performance skills, or performance patterns in order for the client to "[engage] in occupation to support participation" (AOTA, 2002, p. 615) as the ultimate goal. To help clients perform occupations and activities in ADLs, IADLs, work, education, play, and social participation, a combination of intervention approaches is normally required.

Five major intervention approaches may be used singly or in combination, depending on the client's initial and changing needs during intervention. Table 3.7 lists criteria for each intervention approach to indicate how occupational therapists make decisions regarding the selection of an intervention approach. Examples of how these intervention approaches may be successfully interwoven within a single intervention plan are provided later in this guide.

Regardless of the approach used to help clients perform occupations, occupational therapy practitioners use therapeutic teaching as an aspect of each approach (Table 3.8).

Create, Promote (Health Promotion)

Health promotion is defined as "an intervention approach that does not assume a disability is present or that any factors would interfere with per-

Table 3.7. Occupational Therapy Intervention Approaches

Approach	Focus of Intervention	Example
Create, promote (health promotion)	Performance skills	Create a parenting skills training class for first-time parents to increase their knowledge of child development, including the benefits of coregulation, nonverbal dialog, and sensory motorplay.
	Performance patterns	Promote with healthy persons their handling of stress by facilitating time use routines.
	Context(s)	Develop a variety of equipment available at public playgrounds to promote a diversity of sensory play experiences.
	Activity demands	Promote the establishment of sufficient space to allow senior residents to participate in congregate cooking.
	Client factors (body structures, function)	Promote increased endurance in schoolchildren by having them ride bicycles, using helmets and safe riding paths, as a part of an after-school program.
Establish, restore (remediation, restoration)	Performance skills	Improve coping needed for workplace demands by developing assertiveness skills.
	Performance patterns	Establish morning routines needed to arrive at school or work on time.
	Client factors (body structures, function)	Restore the range of motion needed for play activities.
Maintain	Performance skills	Maintain the cognitive skills to organize tools by providing a tool outline painted on a pegboard.
	Performance patterns	Maintain appropriate medication schedule by providing a timer.
	Context(s)	Maintain safe and independent access for people with low vision by providing increased hallway lighting.
	Activity demands	Maintain independent gardening for people with arthritic hands by providing tools with modified grips.
	Client factors (body structures, function)	Maintain upper-extremity muscle strength for independent wheelchair mobility by developing an exercise program.
Modify/compensate	Context(s)	Modify holiday celebrations in the community to support the coping skills related to sobriety by excluding alcohol.
	Activity demands	Modify office equipment (e.g., chair, computer station) to support individual employee body function and performance skill abilities.
	Performance patterns	Modify daily routines to provide consistency and predictability to support a person's cognitive skill ability.
Prevent (disability prevention)	Performance skills	Prevent poor posture when sitting for prolonged periods by having the person learn to use a chair with proper back support.
	Performance patterns	Organize a schedule of healthy daily activities that excludes substance use activities in order to remain drug free.
	Context(s)	Prevent social isolation by suggesting organizations that sponsor after-work group activities.
	Activity demands	Prevent back injury by providing instruction in proper lifting techniques.
	Client factors (body structures, function)	Prevent increased blood pressure during homemaking activities by learning to monitor blood pressure in a cardiac exercise program.

Note. Modified from AOTA (2002), p. 627.

Table 3.8. Teaching as Core to All Approaches

Source	
Therapeutic Teaching Process (Berkeland & Flinn, 2005)	**Examples of Therapeutic Teaching** (Holm, Santangelo, Fromuth, Brown, & Walter, 2000; Peterson & Nelson, 2003; Toglia, 2005; Trombly & Ma, 2002)
Teaching Strategies	

• Determine the characteristics of the learner.
• Identify learning needs.
• Set learning goals.
• Select methods for teaching based on learning styles, such as auditory, visual, or kinesthetic ways to facilitate learning.
• Assess the learning environment.
• Apply evidence-based learning tools unique to the situation, such as
  – Motor learning (organization of practice and feedback to enhance the learning of motor tasks),
  – Errorless learning (use of cues and direction to prevent errors in novel tasks for those with significant cognitive deficits),
  – Attentional focusing (use of externally focused information vs. internally focused information to learn motor tasks),
  – Scaffolding (breaking tasks down into a hierarchy of skills), and
  – Self-monitoring (metacognitive skills to enhance self-awareness).
• Evaluate learning.
• Examine instructor characteristics and style.
	• Match training strategies with the learning capacity of the person.
	• Grade the complexity of what is to be learned.
	• Integrate new learning with previous knowledge.
	• Incorporate practice of activities chosen by the person, repetition, and methods for transfer to a variety of occupations within multiple contexts.
	• Provide training in the use of activity, activity objects, and contextual and environmental modifications.
	• Provide feedback for altering performance.
	• Reinforce correct performance.
	• Incorporate new learning into habits.

formance.... designed to provide enriched contextual and activity experiences that will enhance performance...." (AOTA, 2002, p. 627). Occupational therapy practitioners use three main approaches to promote health and well-being (Wilcock, 2003, 2005):

1. Enable "all people to achieve their fullest health potential" (Wilcock, 2003, p. 42):
   • Target equity of opportunities and resources for participation in healthy occupations and activities
   • Reduce health disparities resulting from occupational deprivation or imbalance
   • Develop personal skills of others in the health-promoting effects of participation in occupations and activities.

2. Mediate "among differing interests in society toward the pursuit of health" (Wilcock, 2003, p. 42):
   • Reorient health services toward the importance of participation in occupations and activities as a vital health promotion strategy
   • Redirect public priorities to enhancing participation in occupations and activities as an aspect of health promotion policy.

3. Advocate with the belief that "health is a major resource for social and economic development, and personal quality of life" (Wilcock, 2003, p. 42):
   • Create supportive environments that access information, life skills, and opportunities for making healthy occupational choices

- Reduce environmental and activity conditions harmful to health.

Establish, Restore (Remediation, Restoration)
Establishment or *restoration* is an intervention approach designed to change client factors and to establish or restore a skill or ability (AOTA, 2002). The *International Classification of Functioning, Disability, and Health* (ICF; WHO, 2001) categories of body structures and functions targeted for remediation and restoration are those necessary for performing desired occupations and activities. In the case of children, those capacities are established because of impaired or slowed development. Specific criteria guide the occupational therapist in selecting remediation and restoration as an approach to intervention (Holm et al., 2003; see Exhibit 3.5).

Appendix G provides the procedural terminology commonly used within the medical model for establishment and restoration. Procedural terminology is important for communicating with third-party payers.

Occupational therapy practitioners use remediation and restoration approaches to prepare the client for more active changes in occupational performance. Many remediation and restoration strategies enable the client to experience reduced pain, reductions in impairments of body structure

---

Exhibit 3.5. Criteria for Remediation and Restoration Approach

An expectation for
- Significantly reducing impairments of body structure and function to
  - Prevent further activity limitations and participation restrictions and
  - Resolve activity limitations or increase participation in occupations and activities;
- Learning new performance skills and patterns;
- Slowing declines in impairments of body structure and function and in occupational performance;
- Maintaining or improving quality of life; and
- Having a context or environment supportive of the time needed for this approach.

---

and function, and improvements in performance skills and patterns. The remediation and restoration approach uses preparatory methods, a type of occupational therapy intervention discussed later in this guide (see p. 44).

Remediation and restoration of body structure and function and of performance skills and patterns are expected to improve occupational performance. As suggested by current motor learning research, however, changes in impairments, skills, and patterns need to transfer to the performance of occupations and activities in the natural context and environment (Shumway-Cook & Woollacott, 2001). By focusing on the transfer of performance skills and patterns and body functioning to the performance of occupations and activities, occupational therapy practitioners acknowledge that linear relationships among impairments, activity limitations, and participation restrictions typically do not exist. Simply expecting improvements in body function to automatically produce change in occupational performance without actually addressing performance in occupations targeted in the intervention plan is inappropriate. The relationships among the *ICF* levels of functioning (WHO, 2001) are complex and are affected by many factors in addition to changes in body functioning or improvements in performance skills and patterns.

Maintain
The intervention approach of *maintain* is "designed to provide the supports that will allow clients to preserve their performance capabilities. ..." (AOTA, 2002, p. 627). Lack of maintain approaches in intervention often results in decreased performance in occupations over time. An example of the maintain approach would be having the client perform exercises to slow declines in occupational performance and to reduce the loss of strength, joint mobility, and functional mobility related to the progressive declines associated with Parkinson's disease. Specific criteria indicate when the maintain approach is an aspect of skilled occupational therapy intervention (Moyers & Christiansen, 2004; see Exhibit 3.6).

Exhibit 3.6. Criteria for Maintain Approach

A need to

- Ensure that the client does not lose current levels of occupational performance;
- Ensure that improvements in occupational performance remain once therapy is withdrawn;
- Slow the anticipated loss of occupational performance with a progressive condition;
- Hold the client accountable for following therapeutic recommendations;
- Train the client how to use therapeutic strategies targeting impairments (e.g., exercise routines or splinting schedules) or how to make activity and environmental modifications (e.g., simplifying activity procedures or adding safety devices in the kitchen and bathroom); and
- Retrain the client with "booster sessions" because of gradual degradation of body functioning, performance skills, and performance patterns.

Modify and Compensate

The intervention approach of *modification and compensation* focuses on revising the context and environment or the activity demands to allow the performance of occupations. For example, compensatory techniques, such as reducing features of the context and environment to improve the client's ability to focus on a particular occupation or activity (AOTA, 2002, p. 627), are effective strategies for enhancing participation. Modification becomes the necessary approach to ensuring occupational performance when intervention directed at performance skills and patterns and at client factors will not accomplish improved performance. Specific criteria indicate the need for the modification and compensation approach (Exhibit 3.7).

Revise the Context and Environment

The *context* and *environment* are defined as the variety of interrelated conditions within and surrounding the client that influence occupational performance. They include cultural, physical, social, personal, temporal, and virtual surroundings.

The extent of changes in the physical context and environment can range from architectural design and new construction to slight modifications to existing structures or objects to strategically

adding assistive devices and technology. Often the occupational therapy practitioner helps reduce costs because simpler modifications may be able to accomplish the same benefit as more elaborately designed modifications. For example, rather than suggest lowering all the kitchen cabinets to accommodate a client in a wheelchair, the occupational therapist or occupational therapy assistant may recommend lowering only a strategically placed work area in the kitchen and rearranging kitchen tools and supplies to promote ease in reaching them from chair height. This approach is especially important because other members of the family, who represent the social context and environment, also need to use the kitchen.

Making revisions in one aspect of the context and environment often requires making modifications or understanding their impact on other aspects of the context. In the example above, revising the structure of the kitchen (physical context) requires adjustment by family members and others (social context) who use the kitchen. Conflicts may arise because of differing beliefs (cultural context) of family members regarding the use of modifications. Performance of an occupation and activity has unique meaning for people

Exhibit 3.7. Criteria for Modification and Compensation Approach

- Expectation for little change in impairments and in performance skills and patterns
- Limited time for intervention
- Preference of person and family, relevant others, or caregivers
- Residual impairments in body structure and function, and performance skills and patterns
- Need for immediate success in occupational performance to sustain motivation for remediation
- Activity limitations and participation restrictions interfere with occupational performance
- Problems of safety, adequacy, and quality during occupational performance
- Existence of remaining occupational performance capabilities that can be enhanced
- Psychological acceptance of the modification.

at different ages (personal context) or stages of life. Use of a modified kitchen may negatively affect one person because the meaning of the modification may signal loss of ability, whereas to another person the modification indicates renewed ability.

Another important aspect of the context and environment is the social context and the need for family and caregiver education. Family members, relevant others, and caregivers need education about how the disorder or injury affects the performance of the client in occupations and activities. The family members and relevant others may need assistance in coping with the changes the disorder and impairments have created in family life. They also benefit from learning how to help the client develop improved body functioning and performance skills and patterns along with ways to help the client enhance participation in important life activities. Collaboration with the family and relevant others is vital to ensure that intervention not only addresses the needs of the client but also considers what the family members or caregivers require to adequately help or supervise the client during occupational performance (Exhibit 3.8). Support from the family or relevant others is important for maintaining the client in the community,

> ### Exhibit 3.8. Collaboration With the Family and Relevant Others
>
> *Occupational therapy practitioners work with family members, relevant others, and caregivers by*
>
> - Teaching how to provide the appropriate level of assistance or supervision for safety;
> - Training in specific, nonskilled strategies designed to maintain gains achieved;
> - Recommending assistive devices and activity and environmental modifications to aid the family, relevant others, and caregivers in providing assistance;
> - Recommending community resources to support the family, relevant others, and caregivers; and
> - Promoting healthy occupational performance of the family, relevant others, and caregivers to ensure the client receives quality care.

thereby avoiding institutionalized forms of care. Table 3.9 presents sample intervention goals for the family and relevant others.

Revise the Activity Demands

The *activity demands* are the "aspects of an activity, which include the objects and their properties, space demands, social demands, sequencing and timing, required actions, and required underlying body functions and body structures needed to carry out the activity" (AOTA, 2002, p. 624).

Table 3.9. Sample Caregiver-Related Intervention Goals

Activity Category	Client Focus of Intervention	Goal Focus on Occupational Performance
Feeding	Activity modification to support sensory functions	The mother will demonstrate the use of calming and positioning techniques to ensure the baby's comfort and safety during breastfeeding.
Functional mobility	Activity and environmental modifications to support residual motor skills	Client's mother will demonstrate proper body mechanics and a safe technique while assisting her son with a standing-pivot transfer to get into bed from the wheelchair.
Personal hygiene and grooming	Activity and environmental modifications to support residual cognitive skills	Caregiver will provide cognitive cuing of one-step verbal directions in order for the client to comb hair and apply makeup with moderate assistance.
Meal preparation and cleanup	Activity and environmental modification to support performance pattern change	The client, with moderate assistance from spouse, will remove all alcohol and drugs from the meal preparation area and will involve a new routine—such as listening to music, monitoring the news on TV, or talking with the children—during daily meal preparation.

The occupational therapy practitioner may *alter an activity object* or its properties used in the performance of occupations by modifying commonly used objects or by recommending object substitutions. For example, providing built-up handles for silverware and tools to counteract lack of grip strength or joint mobility may sufficiently change the activity demands to improve performance in eating and working. Wearing shoes with hook-and-loop fasteners or choosing to wear a slip-on-style shoe may improve the occupation of dressing for someone with motor-skills problems of coordination. In both cases, clients ultimately regain their participation in chosen occupations.

Another method of altering activity objects includes the replacement of commonly used activity objects with objects specifically designed to accommodate impairments in body structure and function and in performance skills. Such objects are referred to as *assistive devices* and *assistive technology*. They span the continuum from basic assistive technology devices (e.g., some ADL devices) to complex or high-tech assistive technology devices (e.g., voice-activated computer systems that interface with a power wheelchair system). Table 3.10 provides examples of assistive devices and assistive technology. Occupational therapy practitioners not only recommend assistive devices and assistive technology but also address the contextual and environmental issues related to the use of the equipment, such as degree of acceptance, social response, loss or gain of roles, level of burden, freedom, and spontaneity in occupational performance (Barker, Reid, & Cott, 2004).

Table 3.10. Examples of Modifications of the Physical Context Through the Use of Assistive Devices and Assistive Technology

Category	Modifications	Category	Modifications
Communication	Modified writing device Computer wrist rests, mouse rests Computer key guards Mouth stick Augmentative communication device Speaker phones Phone headsets	Personal hygiene and grooming	Universal cuff Adapted handles Adapted razors Skin inspection mirror
Dressing	Dressing stick Reachers Extended shoe horn Hook-and-loop closures for clothing Elastic shoelaces Clothes with elastic waistbands Slip-on shoes	Bathing, showering	Grab bars Bath mitts Handheld shower Tub transfer bench Shower commode chair
		Toilet hygiene	Toilet safety frame Bedside commode Bowel training device Bladder control device
Education and work	Modified scissors Pencil grips Slant boards Wrist splint	Mobility Community mobility/ social participation	Modified car seats Automobile hand controls Modified van Taxi or van for the handicapped
Feeding, eating	Modified nipples, bottles Plate guard Modified utensils Modified cups/straws Mobile arm support orthotic	Functional mobility	Wheelchair Slide board Adapted strollers Positioning systems Powered mobility devices
Health management and maintenance	Medication organizer Sample menu plans Modified fitness equipment	Play/leisure	Switch-operated toys Adapted recreation equipment Hand orthotic for grasp of toys
Home establishment or management	Nonskid pad Cutting board Rocker knife Environmental control devices		

The occupational therapy practitioner recognizes that the altering of activity objects used for occupational performance is complex because the alteration may require changes in the activity space, social demands, sequence and timing, required actions, and body functions and structures normally associated with the occupation. For example, use of a wheelchair (to replace walking) at home requires sufficient space to maneuver, cooperation by other family members or relevant others, a specific sequence of steps for correct and safe use, and the development of specific actions with the body. Thus, making a change in one aspect of the activity demand necessarily requires instituting many additional changes.

The complexity of object modification or substitution requires the skills and knowledge of the occupational therapy practitioner to avoid expensive and useless purchases as well as to avoid the development of impairments or safety hazards from improper use. The introduction of assistive devices and assistive technology may radically alter the activity because the new object may make different demands on the body structure and function. The features of the replacement activity object, such as weight and length of the object, may determine whether the new equipment will create problems for the body structure with repetitive use. Additionally, when the replacement object is complex, a high level of cognitive skill is required to learn how to operate it. If the assistive device or assistive technology greatly alters the activity, the success of object modification depends on intact mental functions and cognitive skills for learning how to use the object, when to use the object, and conditions under which use of the object is safe.

Altering sequence, timing, and required actions involves teaching the client new, more efficient, and more effective ways to complete the occupation and activity that more closely correspond with his or her remaining capacities and that do not require use of body structure and function or performance skills and patterns in which the client is deficient. For an occupational therapy practitioner to successfully teach new activity methods, certain requirements must be met (Exhibit 3.9).

Another method of changing the activity demands to improve occupational performance is to *choose a substitute strategy* for completing an activity. For example, rather than driving, the client may take a taxi or a handicap van. Instead of cleaning the house or completing ADL tasks independently, the client may have the resources to hire a maid or a personal attendant. In this way, energy may be conserved for more valued occupations and activities. Hiring assistants, however, could require activity adjustments related to social demands such that modifications in the mental functions (body functions) and cognitive and communication and interaction skills are needed for the client to make the multiple decisions involved in hiring and communicating with an assistant. Using other substitute activity strategies, such as performing the activity in an entirely new manner, may mandate revisions in the objects used and in the manner in which the new objects are used.

Table 3.11 gives examples of how occupational therapy practitioners support the client's participation through revisions of the context or the activity demands.

Prevent (Disability Prevention)
In *disability prevention,* occupational therapy practitioners focus on "[preventing] the occurrence or evolution of barriers to performance" (AOTA, 2002, p. 627). In preventing those barriers, interventions may involve client factors, performance skills or

---

Exhibit 3.9. Client Requirements for Altering Sequence, Timing, and Required Actions of Occupations and Activities

- Adequate learning capacity
- Time for practice
- Motivation by the client, family, relevant others, or caregivers to learn and apply new activity methods
- Supervision of practice from family, relevant others, or caregivers
- Context and environment supportive of activity method modifications
- Activity method modification requiring little new learning.

Table 3.11. Revisions to Context and Activity Demands

Revising the Context or Environment			Revising the Activity Demands		
Aspect of Context or Environment	Modification	Occupational Performance	Aspect of Activity Demand	Modification	Occupational Performance
Physical	Moving well-used kitchen items into cupboards within reach of homemaker	Homemaker can use less energy and maintain balance during meal preparation	Objects and their properties	Increasing the diameter of handles	Carpenter can grasp hammer despite limitations in gripping
Social and cultural	Replacing alcoholic beverages with nonalcoholic beverages for holiday celebrations	Client can engage in safe and responsible social participation with peers during holiday party	Space demands	Purchasing a laptop computer to replace desk model	Student can access voice-activated software at any location
Personal	Getting a college degree in computer technology	Client can find desired employment regardless of quadriplegia	Social demands	Consulting with supervisor to reduce the number of people involved in work project	Worker can contribute to project without getting distracted
Temporal	Using calendar as an organizational tool	Student can attend college classes independently despite impaired cognitive skills in time management	Sequence and timing	Placing affected arm in sleeve first	Person can put on shirt despite stroke
Virtual	Using telecommunication device	Worker with impaired hearing can communicate with employer	Required actions	Using palm to open jar	Homemaker can open jars without stress to finger joints
			Required body functions	Enlarging print on written documents	Student can read required text for school despite low vision
			Required body structures	Using a tenodesis orthotic	Person with quadriplegia can grasp objects despite loss of hand use

patterns, context, or activity demands. Primary prevention focuses on interventions for clients potentially at risk for developing barriers to occupational performance (Epstein & Jaffe, 2003). Occupational therapy practitioners recommend tasks and activities associated with occupations that are conducive to preventing health problems. For example, occupational therapy practitioners may recommend specific toys for children that facilitate development of particular performance skills and patterns.

Secondary prevention focuses on early identification and intervention for clients who have been identified as having risks to occupational performance (Epstein, & Jaffe, 2003). For individuals or populations at risk, the occupational therapy practitioner recommends safer ways to perform activities. For example, to prevent barriers in performance of a work occupation because of the risk for developing cumulative trauma with computer use, the occupational therapy practitioner may ask the worker to take a break at least every half hour from keyboarding to perform a different activity. Stretches and flexibility exercises every 2 hours may be instituted (altering the sequence and timing, requiring new actions with body structures). With regard to objects and their properties, the occupational therapy practitioner may suggest an office chair for better posture and ergonomically designed keyboards.

Tertiary prevention interventions are used with clients who already have activity limitations, impairments, or participation restrictions (Epstein & Jaffe, 2003). This prevention strategy is used to avoid further loss in abilities to perform valued occupations. For example, a client with a spinal cord injury who depends on a wheelchair for mobility also must understand the new activity demands on body structures (arms and shoulders) caused by propelling the wheelchair. The occupational therapy practitioner may employ interventions to alter the activity demands through education or improve capacity through exercise. Similarly, the client who has major depression may be at risk for suicidal thoughts when he or she encounters barriers in the performance of valued occupations. The occupational therapy practitioner teaches coping, stress management, and problem-solving skills as strategies to prevent future suicidal ideation.

Integration of Intervention Approaches

Thus far, this guide has described intervention as involving creation or promotion, establishment or restoration, maintenance, modification, and prevention as though the interventions are instituted individually. In practice, they are interwoven throughout the intervention process and often are used in various combinations according to the needs of the client, family, relevant others, or caregivers. Tables 3.12, 3.13, and 3.14 provide examples of integration of the intervention approaches and techniques within a single intervention plan. These examples do not imply that an intervention plan must include all approaches. For the sake of brevity, the examples focus on one occupational area performance problem, even though the occupational therapy practitioner would address several areas according to the priorities of the client. When possible, the intervention methods are described in the tables according to the procedural terminology used to communicate with third-party payers (Appendix G).

Intervention Implementation

The purpose of intervention implementation is to put the intervention plan into action, a process that involves a skilled occupational therapy process for effecting change in the client's occupational performance and participation in community. "Intervention implementation is a collaborative process between the person and the occupational therapist and the occupational therapy assistant" (AOTA, 2002, p. 618). The focus of intervention is on changing the interrelated and dynamic factors of contexts and environment, activity demands, client factors, performance skills, and performance patterns. Determining how the client's occupational performance responds to changes in those factors is a necessary aspect of intervention implementation.

Intervention implementation includes the following steps (AOTA, 2002):
1. Determine and carry out the type of occupational therapy intervention or interventions to be used.
   - Therapeutic use of self
   - Therapeutic use of occupations or activities
     - Occupation-based activity
     - Purposeful activity
     - Preparatory methods

Table 3.12. Integration of Intervention Approaches: 68-Year-Old Man

Occupational Profile: Client is a 68-year-old man who sustained a head injury in a car accident while driving to the grocery store. Client is retired and lives with his wife.

Analysis of Occupational Performance: Barriers in performance skills and patterns because of impaired body functions such as arm and hand mobility and strength, inability to adjust to activity demands, inability to participate in the physical and social contexts and environments for occupational performance.

Occupational Performance Problem in Area of Occupation	Occupational Performance Goals	Intervention Approaches	Type of Intervention	Outcomes Resulting in Engagement in Occupation to Support Participation
Dressing	To participate in social activities with his wife	Restore neuromusculo-skeletal functions in arms and hands	Preparatory exercise for restoring motion and strength	Regains use of arms and hands to dress appropriately for social activity
Personal hygiene and grooming	To perform volunteer duties at local hospital	Modify small objects for easier and safer grasp, such as using electric shaver rather than straight razor	Modifying the activity demand	Enhanced quality of life
Health maintenance	To take responsibility for implementing a healthy lifestyle	Create, promote routines for nutrition, medication management, and fitness	Purposeful activity to institute new performance patterns	Health and wellness

Table 3.13. Integration of Intervention Approaches: 7-Year-Old Boy

Occupational Profile: Client is a 7-year-old boy who is in the first grade. He has cerebral palsy and lives with his parents.

Analysis of Occupational Performance: Barriers in performing activities at school, such as writing and walking to class because of impaired body functions; impaired social participation due to compromised ability to relate to peers; problems in completing activities of daily living in preparation for going to school.

Occupational Performance Problem in Area of Occupation	Occupational Performance Goals	Intervention Approaches	Type of Intervention	Outcomes Resulting in Engagement in Occupation to Support Participation
Play and formal educational participation	To participate in school and extracurricular activities with peers	Modify the context, such as by collaborating with teachers to adapt the playground and classroom	Occupation-based activity	Role competence as student
Personal hygiene, grooming, and dressing	To prepare self for school and other community activities	Modify objects such as adding Velcro closures for clothing and wider handles for grasping	Compensating for or modifying the activity demands	Client satisfaction
Health maintenance	To participate in community activities as client ages	Create, promote routines for fitness	Preparatory exercise for maintaining motion and strength	Health and wellness

Table 3.14. Integration of Intervention Approaches: Workplace

Occupational Profile: Client is the leader of a safety management team for a local industry and is concerned about the health and wellness of the workforce.

Analysis of Occupational Performance: Barriers to performance in work include stress to body structures due to activity demands, objects that place body structures in compromised postures, performance patterns that create an imbalance of work and rest, and lack of knowledge of similar risk factors in the home context.

Occupational Performance Problem in Area of Occupation	Occupational Performance Goals	Intervention Approaches	Type of Intervention	Outcomes Resulting in Engagement in Occupation to Support Participation
Job performance at work	To participate safely at work	Teach proper posture and lifting to workers and managers	Education process	Role competence as worker
	To reduce injuries at work	Suggest alternative spacing, location, and placement of work objects to reduce stress to body structures	Consultation process	Client satisfaction

- Consultation process
- Education process.

2. Monitor the client's response to interventions using ongoing assessment and reassessment.

Therapeutic use of self refers to the ability to interact with the client in such a way as to gain insights and make judgments as to the client's performance of occupations in response to the occupational therapy practitioner's use of his or her own personality during the occupational therapy process (AOTA, 2002). Therapeutic use of occupations and activities includes the following: *Occupation-based activities* involve intervention focusing on such ADLs or IADLs as dressing prior to going to work or assembling schoolbooks prior to leaving for school. *Purposeful activities* could include simulating handwriting movement requirements or rehearsing a dialogue for assertively interacting with a difficult person at work. *Preparatory methods,* such as exercises or the use of a splint to reduce numbness or pain, are used during intervention as prerequisites to performance in occupations. *Consultation* is an intervention in which the occupational therapy practitioner provides services indirectly and the client accepts responsibility for the actual implementation of the recommendations and the outcomes related to the recommendations. *Education* includes teaching about performance of occupations, but it may or may not require actual performance by the client (AOTA, 2002).

Occupations

The hallmark of occupational therapy intervention is the use of activities meaningful to the client to ensure performance in desired occupations. The activities and occupations chosen as part of the intervention plan are selected with the client to reflect the client's unique occupational profile and occupational history. The principles of occupations make them particularly appropriate and valuable for occupational therapy practitioners as a way to improve occupational performance and health.

Table 3.15 explains the principles of occupations and offers examples of their use in intervention. The research listed in Appendix C supports the use of occupations in intervention.

Individual vs. Group Intervention

Intervention may be provided on an individual basis or within groups (e.g., a family or a class of students; see Table 3.16).

Table 3.15. Principles of Occupations That Support Their Value and Use in Intervention

Principle	Explanation	Example
Occupations and activities act as the therapeutic change agent to *remediate* or *restore*.	People have the potential to improve performance skills, patterns (habits, routines, and rituals), and body functions.	A homemaker who has impairments and problems in motor skills resulting from a stroke benefits more from working in the actual occupation of preparing meals in conjunction with exercises to increase her range of motion, muscle strength, and coordination as opposed to solely using exercise equipment and objects simulating the motor actions of the activity (Gasser-Wieland & Rice, 2002).
The use of new occupations as interventions provides the means for *establishing* performance skills and for developing habits.	The features of the context and environment may have changed and thus may demand the use of new performance skills and habits for the client to perform successfully.	Women with developmental delays and psychiatric conditions had a reduced rate of inappropriate behaviors and increased rate of socially appropriate behaviors in a new community living arrangement when given positive reinforcement in performing everyday occupations (Holm, Santangelo, Fromuth, Brown, & Walter, 2000).
Valued occupations are *inherently motivating*.	Chosen occupations often are a reflection of what people value and enjoy and thus are more likely to be satisfying.	Older adults were motivated to resume engagement in occupations because of opportunities to reestablish relationships with others during engagement in valued occupations (Chan & Spencer, 2004).
Occupations promote the identification of *values* and *interests*.	Values influence occupational choice. When active in occupations, one experiences pleasure and satisfaction, thus generating interests (Kielhofner, 2002).	Older adults living within their communities rated the three most important activities required for them to remain in their communities as using the telephone, using transportation, and reading; health professionals' list consisted of using the telephone, managing medications, and preparing snacks (Fricke & Unsworth, 2001).
Occupations create opportunities to *practice* performance skills and to *reinforce* performance.	The client must have the opportunity to develop patterns that include the remediated skill in routine daily tasks (Holm, Rogers, & Stone, 2003, p. 477).	Elementary students with learning disabilities and handwriting problems who practiced keyboarding in a training program improved written communication skills for performance at school (Handley-More, Deitz, Billingsley, & Coggins, 2003).
Active engagement in occupations produces *feedback*.	Corrective feedback regarding performance helps the client modify behavior.	A computer system was modified for a person with a head injury to provide an auditory prompt to mark the commencement of each planned activity. "I was just sitting there on the sofa doing something like reading a newspaper, and had completely forgotten the swimming bath, then the computer started to bleep; oh, what had I forgotten now?" (Erikson, Karlsson, Söderström, & Tham, 2004, p. 267).
Engagement in occupations facilitates *mastery* or *competence* in performing daily activities.	Successes motivate further change and continued use and practice of newly learned performance skills during engagement in chosen occupations.	People with severe mental illness developed skills and competence in work and social activities while participating in a supported work setting (Gahnstrom-Strandqvist, Liukko, & Tham, 2003).
Selected occupations promote *participation* with individuals or groups.	Interventions designed to eliminate physical and social barriers increase opportunities for social interaction, leading to increased interaction and sense of control in the context and environment.	Children with impaired performance skills used an adapted powered-mobility riding toy, which increased opportunities for participation with other children and adults during the occupation of play (Deitz, Swinth, & White, 2002).

(Continued)

Table 3.15. Principles of Occupations That Support Their Value and Use in Intervention (Continued)

Principle	Explanation	Example
Through engagement in occupations, people learn to *assume responsibility for their own health and wellness*.	Interventions that focus on improving a client's ability to self-direct change in lifestyle choices can lead to a sense of control.	People with chronic disorders who participated in community-based group services developed responsibility for their own health by empowerment of the group members (Taylor, Braveman, & Hammel, 2004).
Occupations exert a positive influence on *health* and *well-being* (Law, 2002b).	Regardless of the presence of impairments, a person may remain active and engaged in healthy occupations.	People with fibromyalgia who successfully used activity modification strategies to complete daily activities reported positive quality of life and health (Lindberg & Iwarsson, 2002).
Occupations provide the means for people to *adapt* to changing needs and conditions.	A person's capacity for performance is affected by the status of body structures and functions. Permanent loss of capacity necessitates modification of the context and environment and of activity demands.	Patients who had hip fractures demonstrated more efficiency and greater satisfaction in recovering performance skills in daily occupations when modified activity procedures were emphasized (Jackson & Schkade, 2001).
Occupations contribute to the creation and maintenance of *identity* (AOTA, 2002; Christiansen, 1999).	Discovering identity is related to what a person does and to those people with whom they come in contact during daily occupations and activities.	People with injuries to the hand resumed occupations that facilitated resumption of their identity (Chan & Spencer, 2004).
Successful performance in occupation can positively affect *psychological* functioning.	A person's evaluation of performance in occupations and activities influences perceptions about himself or herself.	People recovering from a stroke demonstrated positive views and acceptance of the need for a wheelchair, described opportunities for continuity of previous life activities, maintenance of mobility, and decreased burden on the caregiver (Barker, Reid, & Cott, 2004).
Occupations have unique *meaning* and *purpose* for each person, which influences the quality of performance (AOTA, 2002).	The meaning of occupations refers to the subjective experience one has when engaging in activities.	People recovering from a stroke stood longer when performing personally meaningful tasks (Dolecheck & Schkade, 1999).
Engagement in occupations gives a sense of *satisfaction* and *fulfillment* (AOTA, 2002).	Performance of valued occupations provides for achievement of personal goals in a variety of roles.	Satisfaction through occupations was found when older adults maintained daily routines and engaged in fulfilling occupations (Bontje, Kinebanian, Josephsson, & Tamura, 2004). Goldberg, Brintnell, and Golberg (2002) found a correlation between engagement in meaningful activities and life satisfaction.
Occupations influence how people spend time and *make decisions* (AOTA, 2002).	People occupy time through engagement in activities.	In a study of time use, older people spent most of their time completing activities that were meaningful to them and not necessarily the activities that were necessary for them to remain in the community (Fricke & Unsworth, 2001).

Intervention Review

Review occurs periodically during the implementation of the intervention and includes the following steps (AOTA, 2002, p. 618):

• Collaborative reevaluation of the intervention plan as it relates to achieving targeted outcomes

• Modification of the intervention plan as needed
• Determination of the need for continuation, discontinuation, or referral.

Modification of the intervention plan may be indicated when changes have occurred in client factors, the context, performance skills and patterns,

Table 3.16. Individual vs. Group Intervention

Type of Intervention	Consideration in Its Use
Individual	Learning capacity of the person
	Amount of attention and skill required from the occupational therapy practitioner owing to body structure and function impairments
	Need for privacy
	Need for greater control over the context and environment
	Difficulty or complexity of occupation and activity demands, performance skills and performance patterns
	Inappropriate or dangerous behavior of the person
Group	Developing interpersonal skills
	Engaging in socialization
	Receiving feedback from people experiencing similar conditions
	Being motivated by peer role models
	Learning from other people
	Placing one's own condition into perspective
	Developing group normative behavior for successful performance in shared occupations (e.g., work, study, and leisure groups)

or activity demands. For example, strategies used for proper lifting in a work setting may need to be adjusted following the addition of new equipment. Injury to the neuromusculoskeletal system may result in temporary loss of body functions; recovery of those body functions may require new methods of exercise to regain mobility and strength for occupational performance. In all cases, a thorough intervention review is based on collaboration with the client and the client's achievement of outcomes.

Measurement of Outcomes

Ultimately, occupational therapy intervention achieves engagement in occupation to support health and participation in life. Measurement of outcomes (Table 3.17) begins with the evaluation of the client when outcomes are determined and intervention is implemented, so as to achieve those outcomes. During the intervention, periodic review of progress toward the outcomes may require modification of the types of intervention or the targeted outcomes. Occupational therapy services are no longer needed when outcomes have been achieved. Outcomes include occupational performance, client satisfaction, role competence, adaptation, health and wellness, and quality of life (AOTA, 2002).

Occupational therapy outcomes measurement and reporting reflect a shift in the traditional view of health from one based on mortality rates of a population to one "focused on how people live with health conditions and how the individual can achieve a productive, fulfilling life (Baum & Christiansen, 2005a, p. 527). Occupational therapy practitioners also understand that physical function is an incomplete measure of performance in occupations. Outcomes measures reflect performance as influenced by client factors, context and environment, performance patterns and skills, and activity demands.

Outcomes occur as a result of the implementation of a strategy, intervention, or program. Outcomes measurement has many purposes, as follows:
- To discern the effects of the occupational therapy intervention
- To select the occupational performance problems conducive to intervention
- To choose the best approaches to and types of intervention
- To make decisions about frequency, intensity, and duration of intervention
- To determine the client's progress and results
- To change the therapeutic approach

Table 3.17. Types of Outcomes in Occupational Therapy

Outcome	Definition
Occupational performance	The ability to carry out areas of occupation because of improved or enhanced ability to prevent potential problems from developing
Client satisfaction	The client's perceptions of and feelings about the process and benefits of receiving occupational therapy services
Role competence	The ability to effectively meet the demand of roles (e.g., mother, worker, community volunteer)
Adaptation	Changing in response to a new expectation or demands
Health and wellness	A state of physical, mental, and social well-being, balance, and fitness
Quality of life	A person's dynamic appraisal of life satisfaction, self-concept, health and functioning, and socioeconomic factors

- To communicate intervention progress
- To ascertain the effectiveness of an intervention program offered to a group of clients
- To determine sites of future intervention.

Several relevant outcomes can be measured. Outcomes may relate to targets including body structure and function, activity level or occupational performance, participation in life, quality of life, and utility and cost of services.

The measurement plan depends on the targets of the intervention and whether the occupational therapist is evaluating a client's performance or the success of an entire program, which may involve only occupational therapy or may include an interdisciplinary program of services (Kielhofner, Hammel, Finlayson, Helfrich, & Taylor, 2004). Several key critical reasoning questions are answered with outcomes measures:

- What is the client's level of activity and participation?
- Are there any remaining occupational performance problems?
- Has the client's activity and participation truly changed?
- Has the client's activity and participation changed significantly?

Termination of occupational therapy services may include referral to community resources or other professionals, such as other occupational therapy practitioners with specific expertise. For example, the occupational therapist may recommend transfer from a rehabilitation unit of a hospital to extended care (e.g., skilled nursing), an assisted-living facility, home care, or outpatient rehabilitation services. The therapist also may recommend a referral for vocational assessment or for participation in a community self-help program, such as Alcoholics Anonymous. For children, involvement in community programs may be important, such as activities at the YMCA or those planned by community parks. Measurement of outcomes involves the client and other people integral to the situation, such as family members, other health care providers, teachers or school administrators, attorneys, employers, and the insurance carrier. Depending on the client's progress toward targeted outcomes, additional intervention at a later date may be required (Exhibit 3.10).

In some circumstances, the client will need further occupational therapy because of planned medical interventions that occur in stages (e.g., a series of plastic surgeries after a severe burn; a two-stage tendon repair). The client may need to perform new tasks because of changes in the context and environment, such as a new living situation, workplace, caregiver, or teacher. Changes in client factors may provide opportunities to move the client to a higher level of occupational performance (e.g., going from reliance on assistive technology to conventional use of everyday equipment), from one life or developmental stage to another (e.g., from preschool to school, from work to retirement), from one program to another (e.g., from hospital inpatient to home health), or from one physical context to another (e.g., from a job in one part of a building to one in another part of the building). Finally, new technology may enhance the client's ability to engage in desired occupations; its implementation may require intervention to effect modifications in performance patterns and skills.

Exhibit 3.10. Circumstances Requiring Additional Intervention Through Follow-Up

- Occupational performance improves or regresses.
- Changes in client factors interfere with occupational performance or make new occupational performance possible.
- Changes in the context and environment interfere with occupational performance or are able to support new occupational performance.
- Changes in performance patterns or skills interfere with or are developed for occupational performance.
- Activity demands alter occupational performance.

Who Are Occupational Therapists?

To practice as an occupational therapist, the individual trained in the United States
- Has graduated from an occupational therapy program accredited by the Accreditation Council for Occupational Therapy Education (ACOTE) or predecessor organizations,
- Has successfully completed a period of supervised fieldwork experience required by the accredited occupational therapy program,
- Has passed a nationally recognized entry-level examination for occupational therapists, and
- Fulfills state requirements for licensure, certification, or registration.

Educational Programs for the Occupational Therapist

These include the following:
- Biological, physical, social, and behavioral sciences
- Basic tenets of occupational therapy
- Occupational therapy theoretical perspectives
- Screening and evaluation
- Formulation and implementation of an intervention plan
- Context of service delivery
- Management of occupational therapy services
- Use of research
- Professional ethics, values, and responsibilities.

The fieldwork component of the program is designed to develop competent, entry-level, generalist occupational therapists by providing experience with a variety of clients across the life span and in a variety of settings. Fieldwork is integral to the program's curriculum design and includes an in-depth experience in delivering occupational therapy services to clients, focusing on the application of purposeful and meaningful occupation and/or research, administration, and management of occupational therapy services. The fieldwork experience is designed to promote clinical reasoning and reflective practice, to transmit the values and beliefs that enable ethical practice, and to develop professionalism and competence in career responsibilities.

Who Are Occupational Therapy Assistants?

To practice as an occupational therapy assistant, the individual trained in the United States
- Has graduated from an associate- or certificate-level occupational therapy assistant program accredited by ACOTE or predecessor organizations,
- Has successfully completed a period of supervised fieldwork experience required by the accredited occupational therapy assistant program,
- Has passed a nationally recognized entry-level examination for occupational therapy assistants, and
- Fulfills state requirements for licensure, certification, or registration.

Educational Programs for the Occupational Therapy Assistant

These include the following:
- Biological, physical, social, and behavioral sciences
- Basic tenets of occupational therapy
- Screening and assessment
- Intervention and implementation

- Context of service delivery
- Assistance in management of occupational therapy services
- Use of professional literature
- Professional ethics, values, and responsibilities.

The fieldwork component of the program is designed to develop competent, entry-level, generalist occupational therapy assistants by providing experience with a variety of clients across the life span and in a variety of settings. Fieldwork is integral to the program's curriculum design and includes an in-depth experience in delivering occupational therapy services to clients, focusing on the application of purposeful and meaningful occupation. The fieldwork experience is designed to promote clinical reasoning appropriate to the occupational therapy assistant role, to transmit the values and beliefs that enable ethical practice, and to develop professionalism and competence in career responsibilities.

Regulation of Occupational Therapy Practice

All occupational therapists and occupational therapy assistants must practice under federal and state law. Currently, 50 states, the District of Columbia, Puerto Rico, and Guam have enacted laws regulating the practice of occupational therapy.

Note. The majority of this information is taken from the *Standards for an Accredited Educational Program for the Occupational Therapist* (AOTA, 1999b), *Standards for an Accredited Educational Program for the Occupational Therapy Assistant* (AOTA, 1999c), and *Standards of Practice* (AOTA, 2005c).

Continuing competence is a process involving the examination of current competence and the development of capacity for the future. It is a component of ongoing professional development and lifelong learning. Continuing competence is a dynamic, multidimensional process in which the occupational therapist and occupational therapy assistant develop and maintain the knowledge, performance skills, interpersonal abilities, critical reasoning, and ethical reasoning skills necessary to perform current and future roles and responsibilities within the profession.

Occupational therapists and occupational therapy assistants use these standards to assess, maintain, and document continuing competence. Basic to these standards is the belief that all occupational therapists and occupational therapy assistants share core values and knowledge guiding actions within their roles and responsibilities. The core of occupational therapy involves an understanding of occupation and purposeful activities and their influence on human performance. Occupational therapists and occupational therapy assistants have unique skills in activity analysis and activity synthesis and in critical and ethical reasoning. The profession is based on the values of client-centered holistic intervention and the right of an individual to be self-determining.

Standard 1. Knowledge

Occupational therapists and occupational therapy assistants shall demonstrate understanding and comprehension of the information required for the multiple roles and responsibilities they assume. The individual must demonstrate

- Mastery of the core of occupational therapy as it is applied in the multiple responsibilities assumed;

- Expertise associated with primary responsibilities;
- Integration of relevant evidence, literature, and epidemiological data related to primary responsibilities and to the consumer population(s) served; and
- Integration of current Association documents and legislative, legal, and regulatory issues into practice.

Standard 2. Critical Reasoning

Occupational therapists and occupational therapy assistants shall use reasoning processes to make sound judgments and decisions. The individual must demonstrate

- Deductive and inductive reasoning in making decisions specific to roles and responsibilities;
- Problem-solving skills necessary to carry out responsibilities;
- The ability to analyze occupational performance as influenced by environmental factors;
- The ability to reflect on one's own practice;
- Management and synthesis of information from a variety of sources in support of making decisions; and
- Application of evidence, research findings, and outcome data in making decisions.

Standard 3. Interpersonal Abilities

Occupational therapists and occupational therapy assistants shall develop and maintain their professional relationships with others within the context of their roles and responsibilities. The individual must demonstrate

- Use of effective communication methods that match the abilities, personal factors, learning styles, and therapeutic needs of consumers and others;

- Effective interaction with people from diverse backgrounds;
- Use of feedback from consumers, families, supervisors, and colleagues to modify one's professional behavior;
- Collaboration with consumers, families, and professionals to attain optimal consumer outcomes; and
- The ability to develop and sustain team relationships to meet identified outcomes.

Standard 4. Performance Skills

Occupational therapists and occupational therapy assistants shall demonstrate the expertise, aptitudes, proficiencies, and abilities to competently fulfill their roles and responsibilities. The individual must demonstrate expertise in

- Practice grounded in the core of occupational therapy;
- The therapeutic use of self, the therapeutic use of occupations and activities, the consultation process, and the education process to bring about change;
- Integrating current practice techniques and technologies;
- Updating performance based on current research and literature; and
- Quality improvement processes that prevent practice error and maximize client outcomes.

Standard 5. Ethical Reasoning

Occupational therapists and occupational therapy assistants shall identify, analyze, and clarify ethical issues or dilemmas to make responsible decisions within the changing context of their roles and responsibilities. The individual must demonstrate

- Understanding and adherence to the profession's *Code of Ethics,* other relevant codes of ethics, and applicable laws and regulations;
- The use of ethical principles and the profession's core values to understand complex situations; and
- The integrity to make and defend decisions based on ethical reasoning.

Authors

The Commission on Continuing Competence and Professional Development

Penelope Moyers, EdD, OTR/L, BCMH, FAOTA, *Chairperson*

Jane Case-Smith, EdD, OT/L, BCP, FAOTA

Mary Kay Currie, OT, BCPR

Coralie H. Glantz, OT/L, BCG, FAOTA

Jim Hinojosa, OT, PhD, BCP, FAOTA

Maria Elena E. Louch, OT/L, *AOTA Headquarters Liaison*

for

The Commission on Continuing Competence and Professional Development

Penelope Moyers, EdD, OTR/L, FAOTA, *Chairperson*

Adopted by the Representative Assembly 2005C243
Edited 2006

Appendix C | Evidence-Based Practice Resources

American Occupational Therapy Association (AOTA) Evidence Briefs

(www.aota.org)
- *Attention Deficit/Hyperactivity Disorder*
- *Brain Injury*
- *Cerebral Palsy*
- *Children With Behavioral and Psychosocial Needs*
- *Chronic Pain*
- *Developmental Delay in Young Children*
- *Multiple Sclerosis*
- *Older Adults*
- *Parkinson's Disease*
- *School-Based Interventions*
- *Stroke*
- *Stroke: Focused Questions*
- *Substance Use Disorders.*

AOTA's *Evidence-Based Practice Resource Directory*

(www.aota.org)
- Databases and Internet sites in occupational therapy, rehabilitation, and health outcomes
- Tutorials for acquiring basic and intermediate-level skills to search and interpret the literature relevant to occupational therapy
- National and international evidence-oriented Internet sites posted by universities, government agencies, and private organizations.

Agency for Healthcare Research and Quality

(www.ahrq.gov)
The following series of publications are available:
- *Evidence-Based Practice*
- *Outcomes and Effectiveness*
- *Technology Assessments*
- *Preventive Services*
- *Clinical Practice Guidelines.*

Practice Guidelines

Bates, B., Choi, J., Duncan, P., Glasberg, J. J., Graham, G. D., Katz, R. C., et al. (2005). Veterans Affairs/Department of Defense clinical practice guidelines for the management of adult stroke rehabilitation care: Executive summary. *Stroke, 36,* 2049–2056.

Sanders, S., Harden, N., & Vicente, P. J. (2005). Evidence-based clinical practice. Guidelines for interdisciplinary rehabilitation of chronic non-malignant pain syndrome patients. *Pain Practice, 5,* 303–315.

Note. AOTA is continuing to update its Practice Guidelines series. Visit www.aota.org (click "Books, Products, & CE") for the most up-to-date listings.

Practice Patterns

Korner-Bitensky, N., Bitensky, J., Sofer, S., Man-Son-Hing, M., & Gelinas, I. (2006). Driving evaluation practices of clinicians working in the United States and Canada. *American Journal of Occupational Therapy, 60,* 428–434.

Latham, N. K., Jette, D. U., Coster, W., Richards, L., Smout, R. J., James, R. A., et al. (2006). Occupational therapy activities and intervention techniques for clients with stroke in six rehabilitation hospitals. *American Journal of Occupational Therapy, 60,* 369–378.

National Board for Certification in Occupational Therapy. (2004). A practice analysis study of entry-level occupational therapist registered and certified occupational therapy assistant practice.

OTJR: Occupation, Participation, and Health, 24,
S5–S31.

Spencer, K. C., Turkett, A., Vaughan, R., & Koenig,
S. (2006). School-based practice patterns: A survey of occupational therapists in Colorado.
American Journal of Occupational Therapy, 60,
81–91.

Woodward, S., & Swinth, Y. (2002). Multisensory
approach to handwriting remediation: Perceptions of school-based occupational therapists.
American Journal of Occupational Therapy, 56,
305–312.

Reviewed Research

Research reviewed for *The Guide to Occupational
Therapy Practice* was categorized according to the
following criteria:

Case-Control and Cohort Designs

Observational research designed to assess different
designs characteristics and their associations
(Kazdin, 2003). May include correlational studies
and retrospective designs.

Case Study

An intensive evaluation and report of an individual
participant, which could be a person, organization,
or population (Kazdin, 2003).

Meta-analyses

The outcomes of individual studies are the units of
investigation, which are analyzed using specific sta-
tistical procedures in order to synthesize findings in
an objective manner (Law, 2002b).

Multiple Treatment Designs

Participants are randomly assigned to groups, and
each participant receives the interventions under
investigation. May include crossover and multiple-
treatment counterbalanced designs.

Nonrandomized Trials

Study of intervention with a moderate level of control but without random assignment to groups;
may include within-subject as well as matched-
subjects designs.

Outcomes Research

Outcomes research seeks to understand the end
results of particular health care practices and interventions (Agency for Healthcare Research and
Quality, 2000).

Qualitative Research

Naturalistic inquiry or interpretive research that is
rigorous, scientific, disciplined, and replicable. It
includes several research approaches and traditions,
such as ethnography, phenomenology, and
grounded theory (Kazdin, 2003).

Randomized Design

Study of intervention with controls and with random assignment to groups (Kazdin, 2003).

Single-Case Research

Consists of systematic, repeated measurement of
target behavior of one participant through one or
more baseline and intervention phases. Repeated
measures are taken throughout the intervention
phase, a process that permits cause–effect infer-
ences to be made (Kazdin, 2003).

Systematic Reviews

Based on a comprehensive review of the literature
for the purpose of providing an overview of the
validity of research methods and results for a particular topic (Law, 2002b, p. 99).

Outcomes

Occupational Performance

■ Improvement in activities of daily living, instrumental activities of daily living, education, work,
play, leisure, and social participation

Case-Control and Cohort Designs

Beckley, M. N. (2006). Community participation
following cerebrovascular accident: Impact of
the buffering model of social support. *American
Journal of Occupational Therapy, 60,* 129–135.

Classen, S., Mann, W., Wu, S. S., & Tomita, M. R.
(2004). Relationship of number of medications
to functional status, health, and quality of
life for the frail home-based older adult.

OTJR: Occupation, Participation, and Health, 24, 151–160.

Schmidt Hanson, C., Nabavi, D., & Yuen, H. K. (2001). The effect of sports on level of community integration as reported by persons with spinal cord injury. *American Journal of Occupational Therapy, 55,* 332–338.

Case Studies

Boss, T. M. (2006). Responses to the acquisition and use of power mobility by individuals who have multiple sclerosis and their families. *American Journal of Occupational Therapy, 60,* 348–358.

Earley, D., & Shannon, M. (2006). The use of occupation-based treatment with a person who has shoulder adhesive capsulitis: A case report. *American Journal of Occupational Therapy, 60,* 397–403.

Erhardt, R. P., & Meade, V. (2005). Improving handwriting without teaching handwriting: The consultative clinical reasoning process. *Australian Occupational Therapy Journal, 52,* 199–210.

Gillen, G. (2000). Improving activities of daily living performance in an adult with ataxia. *American Journal of Occupational Therapy, 54,* 89–96.

Gillen, G. (2002). Improving mobility and community access in an adult with ataxia. *American Journal of Occupational Therapy, 56,* 462–466.

Krenek, S. M. (2006). A case report on the collaboration of health care professionals in fitting and training seven Iraqi clients with right wrist disarticulations 9 years' postamputation. *American Journal of Occupational Therapy, 60,* 340–347.

Legault, E., & Rebeiro, K. L. (2001). Occupation as means to mental health: A single case study. *American Journal of Occupational Therapy, 55,* 90–96.

Migliore, A. (2004). Improving dyspnea management in three adults with chronic obstructive pulmonary disease. *American Journal of Occupational Therapy, 58,* 639–646.

Phillips, M. E., Katz, J. A., & Harden, R. N. (2000). The use of nerve blocks in conjunction with occupational therapy for complex regional pain syndrome type I. *American Journal of Occupational Therapy, 54,* 544–549.

Meta-analyses

Baker, N. A., & Tickle-Degnen, L. (2001). The effectiveness of physical, psychological, and function interventions in treating clients with multiple sclerosis: A meta-analysis. *American Journal of Occupational Therapy, 55,* 324–331.

Murphy, S., & Tickle-Degnen, L. (2001). The effectiveness of occupational therapy related treatments for persons with Parkinson's disease: A meta-analytic review. *American Journal of Occupational Therapy, 55,* 385–392.

Walker, M. F., Leonardi-Bee, J., Bath, P., Landhorne, P., Dewey, M., Corr, S., et al. (2004). Individual patient data meta-analysis of randomized control trials of community occupational therapy for stroke patients. *Stroke, 35,* 2226–2232.

Multiple-Treatment Designs

Lee, H. L., Tan, H. K.-L., Ma, H.-I., Tsai, C.-Y., & Liu, Y.-K. (2006). Effectiveness of a work-related stress management program in patients with chronic schizophrenia. *American Journal of Occupational Therapy, 60,* 435–441.

Nonrandomized Designs

Case-Smith, J. (2002). Effectiveness of school-based occupational therapy intervention on handwriting. *American Journal of Occupational Therapy, 56,* 17–25.

Fänge, A., & Iwarsson, S. (2005). Changes in ADL dependence and aspects of usability following housing adaptation—A longitudinal perspective. *American Journal of Occupational Therapy, 59,* 296–304.

Landi, F., Cesari, M., Onder, G., Tafani, A., Zamboni, V., & Cocchi, A. (2006). Effects of an occupational therapy program on functional outcomes in older stroke patients. *Gerontology, 52,* 85–91.

Trombly, C. A., Radomski, M. V., Trexel, C., & Burnett-Smith, S. E. (2002). Occupational therapy and achievement of self-identified goals by adults with acquired brain injury: Phase II. *American Journal of Occupational Therapy, 56,* 489–498.

Outcomes Research

Case-Smith, J. (2000). Effects of occupational therapy services on fine motor and functional performance in preschool children. *American Journal of Occupational Therapy, 54,* 372–380.

Case-Smith, J. (2003). Outcomes in hand rehabilitation using occupational therapy services. *American Journal of Occupational Therapy, 57,* 499–506.

Chen, C. C., Heinemann, A. W., Bode, R. K., Granger, C. V., & Mallinson, T. (2004). Impact of pediatric rehabilitation services on children's functional outcomes. *American Journal of Occupational Therapy, 58,* 44–53.

Frank, G., Fishman, M., Crowley, C., Blair, B., Murphy, S. T., Montoya, J. A., et al. (2001). The New Stories/New Cultures after-school enrichment program: A direct cultural intervention. *American Journal of Occupational Therapy, 55,* 501–508.

Guthrie, P. F., Westphal, L., Dahlman, B., Berg, M., Behnam, K., & Ferrell, D. (2004). A patient lifting intervention for preventing the work-related injuries of nurses. *Work, 22,* 79–88.

Hart, D. L., Tepper, S., & Lieberman, D. (2001). Changes in health status for persons with wrist or hand impairments receiving occupational therapy or physical therapy. *American Journal of Occupational Therapy, 55,* 68–74.

Huebner, R. A., Johnson, K., Bennett, C. M., & Schneck, C. (2003). Community participation and quality of life outcomes after adult traumatic brain injury. *American Journal of Occupational Therapy, 57,* 177–185.

Jackson, J. P., & Schkade, J. K. (2001). Occupational adaptation model versus biomechanical–rehabilitation model in the treatment of patients with hip fractures. *American Journal of Occupational Therapy, 55,* 531–537.

Kiefer, D. E., & Emery, L. J. (2006). Self-care and total knee replacement. *Physical and Occupational Therapy in Geriatrics, 24,* 51–62.

Lavelle, P., & Tomlin, G. S. (2001). Occupational therapy goal achievement for persons with postacute cerebrovascular accident in an on-campus student clinic. *American Journal of Occupational Therapy, 55,* 36–42.

Lysack, C. L., MacNeill, S. E., & Lichtenberg, P. A. (2001). The functional performance of elderly urban African-American women who return home to live alone after medical rehabilitation. *American Journal of Occupational Therapy, 55,* 433–440.

Lysack, C. L., Neufeld, S., Mast, B. T., MacNeill, S. E., & Lichtenberg, P. A. (2003). After rehabilitation: An 18-month follow-up of elderly inner-city women. *American Journal of Occupational Therapy, 57,* 298–306.

Marr, D., & Dimeo, S. B. (2006). Outcomes associated with a summer handwriting course for elementary students. *American Journal of Occupational Therapy, 60,* 10–15.

Oka, M., Otsuka, K., Yokoyama, N., Mintz, J., Hoshino, K., Niwa, S.-I., et al. (2004). An evaluation of a hybrid occupational therapy supported employment program in Japan for persons with schizophrenia. *American Journal of Occupational Therapy, 58,* 466–475.

Qualitative Research Designs

Camp, M. M. (2001). The use of service dogs as an adaptive strategy: A qualitative study. *American Journal of Occupational Therapy, 55,* 509–517.

Chan, S. C. C. (2004). Chronic obstructive pulmonary disease and engagement in occupation. *American Journal of Occupational Therapy, 58,* 408–415.

Chan, J., & Spencer, J. (2004). Adaptation to hand injury: An evolving experience. *American Journal of Occupational Therapy, 58,* 128–139.

Copolillo, A., & Teitelman, J. L. (2005). Acquisition and integration of low vision assistive devices: Understanding the decision-making process of older adults with low vision. *American Journal of Occupational Therapy, 59,* 305–313.

Erikson, A., Karlsson, G., Söderström, K., & Tham, K. (2004). A training apartment with electronic aids to daily living: Lived experiences of persons with brain damage. *American Journal of Occupational Therapy, 58,* 261–271.

Ganstrom-Strandqvist, K., Liukko, A., & Tham, K. (2003). The meaning of the working cooperative for persons with long-term mental illness: A phenomenological study. *American Journal of Occupational Therapy, 57,* 262–272.

Gillot, A. J., Holder-Walls, A., Kurtz, J. R., & Varley, N. C. (2003). Perceptions and experiences of two survivors of stroke who participated in constraint-induced movement therapy home programs. *American Journal of Occupational Therapy, 57,* 139–151.

Kielhofner, G., Braveman, B., Finlayson, M., Paul-Ward, A., Goldbaum, L., & Goldstein, K. (2004). Outcomes of a vocation program for persons with AIDS. *American Journal of Occupational Therapy, 58,* 64–72.

Rebeiro, K. L., Day, D. G., Semeniuk, B., O'Brien, M. C., & Wilson, B. (2001). Northern Initiative for Social Action: An occupation-based mental health program. *American Journal of Occupational Therapy, 55,* 493–500.

Siporin, S., & Lysack, C. (2004). Quality of life and supported employment: A case study of three women with developmental disabilities. *American Journal of Occupational Therapy, 58,* 455–465.

Spencer, J., Hersch, G., Shelton, M., Ripple, J., Spencer, C., Dyer, C. B., et al. (2002). Functional outcomes and daily life activities of African-American elders after hospitalization. *American Journal of Occupational Therapy, 56,* 149–159.

Randomized Designs

Chiu, C. W. Y., & Man, D. W. K. (2004). The effect of training older adults with stroke to use home-based assistive devices. *OTJR: Occupation, Participation, and Health, 24,* 113–120.

Dooley, N. R., & Hinojosa, J. (2004). Improving quality of life for persons with Alzheimer's disease and their family caregivers: Brief occupational therapy intervention. *American Journal of Occupational Therapy, 58,* 561–569.

Ivanoff, D., Sonn, S., & Svensson, E. (2002). A health education program for elderly persons with visual impairments and perceived security in the performance of daily occupations: A randomized study. *American Journal of Occupational Therapy, 56,* 322–330.

Norweg, A. M., Whiteson, J., Malgady, R., Mola, A., & Rey, M. (2005). The effectiveness of different combinations of pulmonary rehabilitation program components: A randomized control trial. *Chest, 128,* 663–672.

Peterson, C. Q., & Nelson, D. L. (2003). Effect of an occupational intervention on printing in children with economic disadvantages. *American Journal of Occupational Therapy, 57,* 152–160.

Shaffer, R. J., Jacokes, L. E., Cassily, J. F., Greenspan, S. I., Tuchman, R. F., & Temmer, P. J., Jr. (2001). Effect of interactive Metronome® training on children with ADHD. *American Journal of Occupational Therapy, 55,* 155–162.

Studenski, S., Duncan, P., Perera, S., Reker, D., Min Lai, S., & Richards, L. (2005). Daily functioning and quality of life in a randomized control trial of therapeutic exercise for subacute stroke survivors. *Stroke, 36,* 1764–1770.

Sung, I., Ryu, J., Pyun, S., Yoo, S., Song, W., & Park, M. (2005). Efficacy of forced-use therapy in hemiplegic cerebral palsy. *Archives of Physical Medicine Rehabilitation, 86,* 2195–2198.

Single-Case Research Designs

Deitz, J., Swinth, Y., & White, O. (2002). Powered mobility and preschoolers with complex developmental delays. *American Journal of Occupational Therapy, 56,* 86–96.

Hällgren, M., & Kottorp, A. (2005). Effects of occupational therapy intervention on activities of daily living and awareness of disability in persons with intellectual disabilities. *Australian Occupational Therapy Journal, 52,* 350–359.

Handley-More, D., Deitz, J., Billingsley, F. F., & Coggins, T. E. (2003). Facilitating written work using computer word processing and word prediction. *American Journal of Occupational Therapy, 57,* 139–151.

Holm, M. B., Santangelo, M. A., Fromuth, D. J., Brown, S. O., & Walter, H. (2000). Effectiveness of everyday occupations for changing client behaviors in a community living arrangement. *American Journal of Occupational Therapy, 54,* 361–371.

Labelle, K.-L., & Mihaildis, A. (2006). The use of automated prompting to facilitate handwashing in persons with dementia. *American Journal of Occupational Therapy, 60*, 442–450.

McGruder, J., Cors, D., Tiernan, A. M., & Tomlin, G. (2003). Weighted wrist cuffs for tremor reduction during eating in adults with static brain lesions. *American Journal of Occupational Therapy, 57*, 507–516.

Schilling, D. L., Washington, K., Billingsley, F. F., & Deitz, J. (2003). Classroom seating for children with attention deficit hyperactivity disorder: Therapy balls versus chairs. *American Journal of Occupational Therapy, 57*, 534–541.

Tanta, K. J., Deitz, J. C., White, O., & Billingsley, F. (2005). The effects of peer-play level on initiations and responses of preschool children with delayed play skills. *American Journal of Occupational Therapy, 59*, 437–445.

Tham, K., Ginsburg, E., Fisher, A. G., & Tegnér, R. (2001). Training to improve awareness of disabilities in clients with unilateral neglect. *American Journal of Occupational Therapy, 55*, 46–54.

Systematic Reviews

Crowther, R., Marshall, M., Bond, G., & Huxley P. (2001). Vocational rehabilitation for people with severe mental illness. *Cochrane Database of Systematic Reviews*, Issue 2, CD003080. DOI: 10.1002/14651858.CD003080.

Guzmán, J., Esmail, R., Karjalainen, K., Malmivaara, A., Irvin, E., & Bombardier, C. (2002). Multidisciplinary bio-psycho-social rehabilitation for chronic low-back pain. *Cochrane Database of Systematic Reviews*, Issue 1, CD000963. DOI: 10.1002/14651858.CD000963.

Karjalainen, K., Malmivaara, A., van Tulder, M., Roine, R., Jauhiainen, M., Hurri, H., et al. (2003). Multidisciplinary biopsychosocial rehabilitation for subacute low-back pain among working-age adults. *Cochrane Database of Systematic Reviews*, Issue 2, CD002193. DOI:10.1002/14651858.CD002193.

Outpatient Service Trialists. (2003). Therapy-based rehabilitation services for stroke patients at home. *Cochrane Database of Systematic Reviews*, Issue 1, CD002925. DOI:10.1002/14651858.CD002925.

Schonstein, E., Kenny, D. T., Keating, J., & Koes, B. W. (2003). Work conditioning, work hardening, and functional restoration for workers with back and neck pain. *Cochrane Database of Systematic Reviews*, Issue 3, CD001822. DOI:10.1002/14651858.CD001822.

Steultjens, E. E. M. J., Bouter, L. L. M., Dekker, J. J., Kuyk, M. M. A. H., Schaardenberg, D. D., & Van den Ende, E. C. H. M. (2004). Occupational therapy for rheumatoid arthritis. *Cochrane Database of Systematic Reviews*, Issue 1, CD003114. DOI: 10.1002/14651858.CD003114.pub2.

Stoffel, V. C., & Moyers, P. A. (2004). An evidence-based and occupational perspective of interventions for persons with substance-use disorders. *American Journal of Occupational Therapy, 56*, 570–586.

Stroke Unit Trialists' Collaboration. (2001). Organised inpatient (stroke unit) care for stroke. *Cochrane Database of Systematic Reviews*, Issue 3, CD000197. DOI:10.1002/14651858.CD000197.

Trombly, C. A., & Ma, H. (2002). A synthesis of the effects of occupational therapy for persons with stroke, part I: Restoration of roles, tasks, and activities. *American Journal of Occupational Therapy, 56*, 250–259.

Turner-Stokes, L., Disler, P. B., Nair, A., & Wade, D. T. (2005). Multi-disciplinary rehabilitation for acquired brain injury in adults of working age. *Cochrane Database of Systematic Reviews*, Issue 3, CD004170. DOI:10.1002/14651858.CD004170.pub2.

■ Underlying factors involving performance skills and patterns and body structure/body function

Case-Control and Cohort Designs

Callinan, N., McPherson, S., Cleaveland, S., Voss, D. G., Rainville, D., & Tokar, N. (2003). Effectiveness of hydroplasty and therapeutic exercise for treatment of frozen shoulder. *Journal of Hand Therapy, 16*, 219–224.

Klein, L. (2003). Early active motion flexor tendon protocol using one splint. *Journal of Hand Therapy, 16,* 199–206.

Case Studies

Earley, D., & Shannon, M. (2006). The use of occupation-based treatment with a person who has shoulder adhesive capsulitis: A case report. *American Journal of Occupational Therapy, 60,* 397–403.

Gillen, G. (2002). Improving mobility and community access in an adult with ataxia. *American Journal of Occupational Therapy, 56,* 462–466.

Hurst, C. M. F., Van de Weyer, S., Smith, C., & Adler, P. M. (2006). Improvements in performance following optometric vision therapy in a child following dyspraxia. *Ophthalmic and Physiological Optics, 26,* 199–210.

Migliore, A. (2004). Improving dyspnea management in three adults with chronic obstructive pulmonary disease. *American Journal of Occupational Therapy, 58,* 639–646.

Nilsson, L. M., & Nyberg, P. J. (2003). Driving to learn: A new concept for training children with profound cognitive disabilities in a powered wheelchair. *American Journal of Occupational Therapy, 57,* 229–233.

Phillips, M. E., Katz, J. A., & Harden, R. N. (2000). The use of nerve blocks in conjunction with occupational therapy for complex regional pain syndrome type I. *American Journal of Occupational Therapy, 54,* 544–549.

Meta-analyses

Baker, N. A., & Tickle-Degnen, L. (2001). The effectiveness of physical, psychological, and function interventions in treating clients with multiple sclerosis: A meta-analysis. *American Journal of Occupational Therapy, 55,* 324–331.

Murphy, S., & Tickle-Degnen, L. (2001). The effectiveness of occupational therapy related treatments for persons with Parkinson's disease: A meta-analytic review. *American Journal of Occupational Therapy, 55,* 385–392.

Multiple-Treatment Designs

Maitra, K. K., Telage, K. M., & Rice, M. S. (2006). Self-speech–induced facilitation of simple reaching movements in persons with stroke. *American Journal of Occupational Therapy, 60,* 146–154.

Vanage, S. M., Gilbertson, K. K., & Mathiowetz, V. (2003). Effects of an energy conservation course on fatigue impact for persons with progressive multiple sclerosis. *American Journal of Occupational Therapy, 57,* 315–323.

Nonrandomized Designs

Dankert, H. L., Davies, P. L., & Gavin, W. L. (2003). Occupational therapy effects on visual–motor skills in preschool children. *American Journal of Occupational Therapy, 57,* 542–549.

Dreiling, D. S., & Bundy, A. C. (2003). A comparison of consultative model and direct–indirect intervention with preschoolers. *American Journal of Occupational Therapy, 57,* 566–569.

Fasoli, S. E., Trombly, C. A., Tickle-Degnen, L., & Verfaellie, M. H. (2002). Effect of instruction on functional reach in persons with and without cerebrovascular accident. *American Journal of Occupational Therapy, 56,* 380–390.

Landi, F., Cesari, M., Onder, G., Tafani, A., Zamboni, V., & Cocchi, A. (2006). Effects of an occupational therapy program on functional outcomes in older stroke patients. *Gerontology, 52,* 85–91.

Smith, S. A., Press, B., Koenig, K. P., & Kinnealey, M. (2005). Effects of sensory integration intervention on self-stimulating and self-injurious behaviors. *American Journal of Occupational Therapy, 59,* 418–425.

Outcomes Research

Case-Smith, J. (2003). Outcomes in hand rehabilitation using occupational therapy services. *American Journal of Occupational Therapy, 57,* 499–506.

Droeze, E. H., & Jonsson, H. (2005). Evaluation of ergonomic interventions to reduce musculoskeletal disorders of dentists in the Netherlands. *Work, 25,* 211–220.

Lavelle, P., & Tomlin, G. S. (2001). Occupational therapy goal achievement for persons with postacute cerebrovascular accident in an on-campus student clinic. *American Journal of Occupational Therapy, 55,* 36–42.

Lysack, C. L., MacNeill, S. E., & Lichtenberg, P. A. (2001). The functional performance of elderly urban African-American women who return home to live alone after medical rehabilitation. *American Journal of Occupational Therapy, 55,* 433–440.

Sharek, P. J., Wayman, K., Lin, E., Strichartz, D., Sentivany-Collins, S., Good, J., et al. (2006). Improved pain management in pediatric postoperative liver transplant patients using parental education and non-pharmacological interventions. *Pediatric Transplantation, 10,* 172–177.

Qualitative Research Designs

Chan, J., & Spencer, J. (2004). Adaptation to hand injury: An evolving experience. *American Journal of Occupational Therapy, 58,* 128–139.

Randomized Designs

Cheng, A. S.-K. (2000). Use of early tactile stimulation in rehabilitation of digital nerve injuries. *American Journal of Occupational Therapy, 54,* 159–165.

Glasgow, C., Wilton, J., & Tooth, L. (2003). Optimal daily total end range time for contracture: Resolution in hand splinting. *Journal of Hand Therapy, 16,* 207–218.

Jarus, T., Shavit, S., & Ratzon, N. (2000). From hand twister to mind twister: Computer–aided treatment in traumatic wrist fracture. *American Journal of Occupational Therapy, 54,* 176–182.

Norweg, A. M., Whiteson, J., Malgady, R., Mola, A., & Rey, M. (2005). The effectiveness of different combinations of pulmonary rehabilitation program components: A randomized control trial. *Chest, 128,* 663–672.

Shaffer, R. J., Jacokes, L. E., Cassily, J. F., Greenspan, S. I., Tuchman, R. F., & Temmer, P. J., Jr. (2001). Effect of interactive Metronome® training on children with ADHD. *American Journal of Occupational Therapy, 55,* 155–162.

Studenski, S., Duncan, P., Perera, S., Reker, D., Min Lai, S., & Richards, L. (2005). Daily functioning and quality of life in a randomized control trial of therapeutic exercise for subacute stroke survivors. *Stroke, 36,* 1764-1770.

Sung, I., Ryu, J., Pyun, S., Yoo, S., Song, W., & Park, M. (2005). Efficacy of forced-use therapy in hemiplegic cerebral palsy. *Archives of Physical Medicine Rehabilitation, 86,* 2195–2198.

Single-Case Research Designs

Deitz, J., Swinth, Y., & White, O. (2002). Powered mobility and preschoolers with complex developmental delays. *American Journal of Occupational Therapy, 56,* 86–96.

Fettel-Daly, D., Bedell, G., & Hinojosa, J. (2001). Effects of a weighted vest on attention to task and self-stimulatory behaviors in preschoolers with pervasive developmental disorders. *American Journal of Occupational Therapy, 55,* 629–640.

Hällgren, M., & Kottorp, A. (2005). Effects of occupational therapy intervention on activities of daily living and awareness of disability in persons with intellectual disabilities. *Australian Occupational Therapy Journal, 52,* 350–359.

Kawahira, K., Shimodozono, M., Etoh, S., & Tanaka, N. (2005). New facilitation exercise using the vestibulo-ocular reflex for opthalmoplegia: Preliminary report. *Clinical Rehabilitation, 19,* 627–634.

McGruder, J., Cors, D., Tiernan, A. M., & Tomlin, G. (2003). Weighted wrist cuffs for tremor reduction during eating in adults with static brain lesions. *American Journal of Occupational Therapy, 57,* 507–516.

Melchert-McKearnan, K., Deitz, J., Engel, J. M., & White, O. (2000). Children with burn injuries: Purposeful activity versus rote exercise. *American Journal of Occupational Therapy, 54,* 381–390.

Tham, K., Ginsburg, E., Fisher, A. G., & Tegnér, R. (2001). Training to improve awareness of disabilities in clients with unilateral neglect. *American Journal of Occupational Therapy, 55,* 46–54.

Systematic Reviews

Bowen, A., Lincoln, N. B., & Dewey, M. (2002). Cognitive rehabilitation for spatial neglect following a stroke. *Cochrane Database of Systematic Reviews,* Issue 2, CD003586. DOI:10.1002/14651858. CD003586.

Dinh-Zarr, T., Goss, C., Heitman, E., Roberts, I., & DiGuiseppi, C. (2004). Interventions for preventing injuries in problem drinkers. *Cochrane Database of Systematic Reviews,* Issue 3, CD001857. DOI:10.1002/14651858.CD001857.pub2.

Guzmán, J., Esmail, R., Karjalainen, K., Malmivaara, A., Irvin, E., & Bombardier, C. (2002). Multidisciplinary bio-psycho-social rehabilitation for chronic low-back pain. *Cochrane Database of Systematic Reviews,* Issue 1, CD000963. DOI: 10.1002/14651858.CD000963.

Han, A., Judd, M. G., Robinson, V. A., Taixiang, W., Tugwell, P., & Wells, G. (2004). Tai chi for treating rheumatoid arthritis. *Cochrane Database of Systematic Reviews,* Issue 3, CD004849. DOI: 10.1002/14651858.CD004849.

Lincoln, N. B., Majid, M. J., & Weyman, N. (2000). Cognitive rehabilitation for attention deficits following stroke. *Cochrane Database of Systematic Reviews,* Issue 4, CD002842. DOI:10.1002/14651858.CD002842.

O'Brien, K., Nixon, S., Glazier, R. H., & Tynan, A. M. (2004). Progressive resistive interventions for adults living with HIV/AIDS. *Cochrane Database of Systematic Reviews,* Issue 4, CD004248. DOI: 10.1002/14651858.CD004248.pub2.

Ostelo, R. W. J. G., van Tudler, M. W., Vlaeyen, J. W. S., Linton, S. J., & Assendelft, W. J. J. (2005). Behavioural treatment for chronic low-back pain. *Cochrane Database of Systematic Reviews,* Issue 1, CD002014. DOI:10.1002/14651858. CD002014.pub2.

Pelland, L., Brosseau, L., Casimiro, L., Robinson, V. A., Tugwell, P., & Wells, G. (2002). Electrical stimulation for the treatment of rheumatoid arthritis. *Cochrane Database of Systematic Reviews,* Issue 2, CD003687. DOI:10.1002/14651858. CD003678.

Rietberg, M. B., Brooks, D., Uitdehaag, B. M. J., & Kwakkel, G. (2004). Exercise therapy for multiple sclerosis. *Cochrane Database of Systematic Reviews,* Issue 3, CD003980. DOI:10.1002/14651858. CD003980.pub2.

Schonstein, E., Kenny, D. T., Keating, J., & Koes, B. W. (2003). Work conditioning, work hardening and functional restoration for workers with back and neck pain. *Cochrane Database of Systematic Reviews,* Issue 3, CD001822. DOI:10.1002/14651858.CD001822.

Steultjens, E. E. M. J., Bouter, L. L. M., Dekker, J. J., Kuyk, M. M. A. H., Schaardenberg, D. D., & Van den Ende, E. C. H. M. (2004). Occupational therapy for rheumatoid arthritis. *Cochrane Database of Systematic Reviews,* Issue 1, CD003114. DOI: 10.1002/14651858.CD003114.pub2.

Stoffel, V. C., & Moyers, P. A. (2004). An evidence-based and occupational perspective of interventions for persons with substance-use disorders. *American Journal of Occupational Therapy, 56,* 570–586.

Trombly, C. A., & Ma, H. (2002). A synthesis of the effects of occupational therapy for persons with stroke, part II: Remediation of impairments. *American Journal of Occupational Therapy, 56,* 250–259.

Van den Ende, C. H. M., Vliet Vlieland, T. P. M., Munneke, M., & Hazes, J. M. W. (1998). Dynamic exercise therapy for treating rheumatoid arthritis. *Cochrane Database of Systematic Reviews,* Issue 4, CD000322. DOI:10.1002/14651858.CD000322.

Wallen, M., & Gillies, D. (2006). Intra-articular steroids and splints/rest for children with juvenile idiopathic arthritis and adults with rheumatoid arthritis. *Cochrane Database of Systematic Reviews,* Issue 1, CD002824. DOI:10.1002/14651858.CD002824.pub2.

Woods, B., Spector, A., Jones, C., Orrell, M., & Davies, S. (2005). Reminiscence therapy for dementia. *Cochrane Database of Systematic Reviews,* Issue 2, CD001120. DOI:10.1002/14651858.CD001120.pub2.

Personal Satisfaction

Case Studies

Migliore, A. (2004). Improving dyspnea management in three adults with chronic obstructive pulmonary disease. *American Journal of Occupational Therapy, 58,* 639–646.

Nonrandomized Designs

Jackson, J. P., & Schkade, J. K. (2001). Occupational adaptation model versus biomechanical–rehabilitation model in the treatment of patients with hip fractures. *American Journal of Occupational Therapy, 55,* 531–537.

Trombly, C. A., Radomski, M. V., Trexel, C., & Burnett-Smith, S. E. (2002). Occupational therapy and achievement of self-identified goals by adults with acquired brain injury: Phase II. *American Journal of Occupational Therapy, 56,* 489–498.

Outcomes Research

Frank, G., Fishman, M., Crowley, C., Blair, B., Murphy, S. T., Montoya, J. A., et al. (2001). The New Stories/New Cultures after-school enrichment program: A direct cultural intervention. *American Journal of Occupational Therapy, 55,* 501–508.

Hart, D. L., Tepper, S., & Lieberman, D. (2001). Changes in health status for persons with wrist or hand impairments receiving occupational therapy or physical therapy. *American Journal of Occupational Therapy, 55,* 68–74.

Huebner, R. A., Johnson, K., Bennett, C. M., & Schneck, C. (2003). Community participation and quality of life outcomes after adult traumatic brain injury. *American Journal of Occupational Therapy, 57,* 177–185.

Qualitative Research Designs

Bontje, P., Kinébanian, A., Josephsson, S., & Tamura, Y. (2004). Occupational adaptation: The experiences of older persons with physical disabilities. *American Journal of Occupational Therapy, 58,* 140–149.

Ganstrom-Strandqvist, K., Liukko, A., & Tham, K. (2003). The meaning of the working cooperative for persons with long-term mental illness: A phenomenological study. *American Journal of Occupational Therapy, 57,* 262–272.

Gillot, A. J., Holder-Walls, A., Kurtz, J. R., & Varley, N. C. (2003). Perceptions and experiences of two survivors of stroke who participated in constraint-induced movement therapy home programs. *American Journal of Occupational Therapy, 57,* 139–151.

Siporin, S., & Lysack, C. (2004). Quality of life and supported employment: A case study of three women with developmental disabilities. *American Journal of Occupational Therapy, 58,* 455–465.

Randomized Designs

Chiu, C. W. Y., & Man, D. W. K. (2004). The effect of training older adults with stroke to use home-based assistive devices. *OTJR: Occupation, Participation, and Health, 24,* 113–120.

VanLeit, B., & Crowe, T. K. (2002). Outcomes of an occupational therapy program for mothers of children with disabilities: Impact on satisfaction with time use and occupational performance. *American Journal of Occupational Therapy, 56,* 402–410.

Systematic Reviews

Han, A., Judd, M. G., Robinson, V. A., Taixiang, W., Tugwell, P., & Wells, G. (2004). Tai chi for treating rheumatoid arthritis. *Cochrane Database of Systematic Reviews,* Issue 3, CD004849. DOI: 10.1002/14651858.CD004849.

Role Competence

Case-Control and Cohort Designs

Schmidt Hanson, C., Nabavi, D., & Yuen, H. K. (2001). The effect of sports on level of community integration as reported by persons with spinal cord injury. *American Journal of Occupational Therapy, 55,* 332–338.

Case Studies

Gillen, G. (2000). Improving activities of daily living performance in an adult with ataxia. *American Journal of Occupational Therapy, 54,* 89–96.

Legault, E., & Rebiro, K. L. (2001). Occupational as means to mental health: A single case study. *American Journal of Occupational Therapy, 55,* 90–96.

Meta-analysis

Baker, N. A., & Tickle-Degnen, L. (2001). The effectiveness of physical, psychological, and function interventions in treating clients with multiple sclerosis: A meta-analysis. *American Journal of Occupational Therapy, 55,* 324–331.

Nonrandomized Designs

Case-Smith, J. (2002). Effectiveness of school-based occupational therapy intervention on handwriting. *American Journal of Occupational Therapy, 56,* 17–25.

Outcome Studies

Guthrie, P. F., Westphal, L., Dahlman, B., Berg, M., Behnam, K., & Ferrell, D. (2004). A patient lifting intervention for preventing the work-related injuries of nurses. *Work, 22,* 79–88.

Marr, D., & Dimeo, S. B. (2006). Outcomes associated with a summer handwriting course for elementary students. *American Journal of Occupational Therapy, 60,* 10–15.

Oka, M., Otsuka, K., Yokoyama, N., Mintz, J., Hoshino, K., Niwa, S.-I., et al. (2004). An evaluation of a hybrid occupational therapy supported employment program in Japan for persons with schizophrenia. *American Journal of Occupational Therapy, 58,* 466–475.

Qualitative Research Designs

Camp, M. M. (2001). The use of service dogs as an adaptive strategy: A qualitative study. *American Journal of Occupational Therapy, 55,* 509–517.

Ganstrom-Strandqvist, K., Liukko, A., & Tham, K. (2003). The meaning of the working cooperative for persons with long-term mental illness: A phenomenological study. *American Journal of Occupational Therapy, 57,* 262–272.

Howie, L., Coulter, M., & Feldman, S. (2004). Crafting the self: Older persons' narratives of occupational identity. *American Journal of Occupational Therapy, 58,* 446–454.

Kielhofner, G., Braveman, B., Finlayson, M., Paul-Ward, A., Goldbaum, L., & Goldstein, K. (2004). Outcomes of a vocation program for persons with AIDS. *American Journal of Occupational Therapy, 58,* 64–72.

Randomized Designs

Peterson, C. Q., & Nelson, D. L. (2003). Effect of an occupational intervention on printing in children with economic disadvantages. *American Journal of Occupational Therapy, 57,* 152–160.

Studenski, S., Duncan, P., Perera, S., Reker, D., Min Lai, S., & Richards, L. (2005). Daily functioning and quality of life in a randomized control trial of therapeutic exercise for subacute stroke survivors. *Stroke, 36,* 1764–1770.

Single-Case Research Designs

Handley-More, D., Deitz, J., Billingsley, F. F., & Coggins, T. E. (2003). Facilitating written work using computer word processing and word prediction. *American Journal of Occupational Therapy, 57,* 139–151.

Schilling, D. L., Washington, K., Billingsley, F. F., & Deitz, J. (2003). Classroom seating for children with attention deficit hyperactivity disorder: Therapy balls versus chairs. *American Journal of Occupational Therapy, 57,* 534–541.

Tanta, K. J., Deitz, J. C., White, O., & Billingsley, F. (2005). The effects of peer-play level on initiations and responses of preschool children with delayed play skills. *American Journal of Occupational Therapy, 59,* 437–445.

Systematic Reviews

Trombly, C. A., & Ma, H. (2002). A synthesis of the effects of occupational therapy for persons with stroke, part I: Restoration of roles, tasks, and activities. *American Journal of Occupational Therapy, 56,* 250–259.

Adaptation

Case Studies

Boss, T. M. (2006). Responses to the acquisition and use of power mobility by individuals who have multiple sclerosis and their families. *American Journal of Occupational Therapy, 60,* 348–358.

Erhardt, R. P., & Meade, V. (2005). Improving handwriting without teaching handwriting: The consultative clinical reasoning process. *Australian Occupational Therapy Journal, 52,* 199–210.

Gillen, G. (2000). Improving activities of daily living performance in an adult with ataxia. *American Journal of Occupational Therapy, 54,* 89–96.

Gillen, G. (2002). Improving mobility and community access in an adult with ataxia. *American Journal of Occupational Therapy, 56,* 462–466.

Migliore, A. (2004). Improving dyspnea management in three adults with chronic obstructive pulmonary disease. *American Journal of Occupational Therapy, 58,* 639–646.

Phillips, M. E., Katz, J. A., & Harden, R. N. (2000). The use of nerve blocks in conjunction with occupational therapy for complex regional pain syndrome type I. *American Journal of Occupational Therapy, 54,* 544–549.

Nonrandomized Designs

Dankert, H. L., Davies, P. L., & Gavin, W. L. (2003). Occupational therapy effects on visual–motor skills in preschool children. *American Journal of Occupational Therapy, 57,* 542–549.

Dreiling, D. S., & Bundy, A. C. (2003). A comparison of consultative model and direct–indirect intervention with preschoolers. *American Journal of Occupational Therapy, 57,* 566–569.

Fänge, A., & Iwarsson, S. (2005). Changes in ADL dependence and aspects of usability following housing adaptation—A longitudinal perspective. *American Journal of Occupational Therapy, 59,* 296–304.

Jackson, J. P., & Schkade, J. K. (2001). Occupational adaptation model versus biomechanical–rehabilitation model in the treatment of patients with hip fractures. *American Journal of Occupational Therapy, 55,* 531–537.

Landi, F., Cesari, M., Onder, G., Tafani, A., Zamboni, V., & Cocchi, A. (2006). Effects of an occupational therapy program on functional outcomes in older stroke patients. *Gerontology, 52,* 85–91.

Trombly, C. A., Radomski, M. V., Trexel, C., & Burnett-Smith, S. E. (2002). Occupational therapy and achievement of self-identified goals by adults with acquired brain injury: Phase II. *American Journal of Occupational Therapy, 56,* 489–498.

Outcomes Research

Droeze, E. H., & Jonsson, H. (2005). Evaluation of ergonomic interventions to reduce musculoskeletal disorders of dentists in the Netherlands. *Work, 25,* 211–220.

Lysack, C. L., MacNeill, S. E., & Lichtenberg, P. A. (2001). The functional performance of elderly urban African-American women who return home to live alone after medical rehabilitation. *American Journal of Occupational Therapy, 55,* 433–440.

Qualitative Research Designs

Bontje, P., Kinébanian, A., Josephsson, S., & Tamura, Y. (2004). Occupational adaptation: The experiences of older persons with physical disabilities. *American Journal of Occupational Therapy, 58,* 140–149.

Camp, M. M. (2001). The use of service dogs as an adaptive strategy: A qualitative study. *American Journal of Occupational Therapy, 55,* 509–517.

Chan, J., & Spencer, J. (2004). Adaptation to hand injury: An evolving experience. *American Journal of Occupational Therapy, 58,* 128–139.

Copolillo, A., & Teitelman, J. L. (2005). Acquisition and integration of low vision assistive devices: Understanding the decision-making process of older adults with low vision. *American Journal of Occupational Therapy, 59,* 305–313.

Dale, L. (2004). Partnering with management to implement ergonomics in the industrial setting. *Work, 22,* 117–124.

Erikson, A. Karlsson, G., Söderström, K., & Tham, K. (2004). A training apartment with electronic aids to daily living: Lived experiences of persons with brain damage. *American Journal of Occupational Therapy, 58,* 261–271.

Gillot, A. J., Holder-Walls, A., Kurtz, J. R., & Varley, N. C. (2003). Perceptions and experiences of two survivors of stroke who participated in constraint-induced movement therapy home programs. *American Journal of Occupational Therapy, 57,* 139–151.

Spencer, J., Hersch, G., Shelton, M., Ripple, J., Spencer, C., Dyer, C. B., et al. (2002). Functional outcomes and daily life activities of African-American elders after hospitalization. *American Journal of Occupational Therapy, 56,* 149–159.

Randomized Designs

Chiu, C. W. Y., & Man, D. W. K. (2004). The effect of training older adults with stroke to use home-based assistive devices. *OTJR: Occupation, Participation, and Health, 24,* 113–120.

Dooley, N. R., & Hinojosa, J. (2004). Improving quality of life for persons with Alzheimer's disease and their family caregivers: Brief occupational therapy intervention. *American Journal of Occupational Therapy, 58,* 561–569.

Gillot, A. J., Holder-Walls, A., Kurtz, J. R., & Varley, N. C. (2003). Perceptions and experiences of two survivors of stroke who participated in constraint-induced movement therapy home programs. *American Journal of Occupational Therapy, 57,* 139–151.

Mathiowetz, V., Finlayson, M. L., Matuska, K. M., Chen, H. Y., & Luo, P. (2005). Randomized control trial of an energy conservation course for persons with multiple sclerosis. *Multiple Sclerosis, 11,* 592–601.

Single-Case Research Designs

McGruder, J., Cors, D., Tiernan, A. M., & Tomlin, G. (2003). Weighted wrist cuffs for tremor reduction during eating in adults with static brain lesions. *American Journal of Occupational Therapy, 57,* 507–516.

Schilling, D. L., Washington, K., Billingsley, F. F., & Deitz, J. (2003). Classroom seating for children with attention deficit hyperactivity disorder: Therapy balls versus chairs. *American Journal of Occupational Therapy, 57,* 534–541.

Tham, K., Ginsburg, E., Fisher, A. G., & Tegnér, R. (2001). Training to improve awareness of disabilities in clients with unilateral neglect. *American Journal of Occupational Therapy, 55,* 46–54.

Systematic Reviews

Gillespie, L. D., Gillespie, W. J., Robertson, M. C., Lamb, S. E., Cumming, R. G., & Rowe, B. H. (2003). Interventions for preventing falls in elderly people. *Cochrane Database of Systematic Reviews,* Issue 4, CD000340. DOI:10.1002/14651858.CD000340.

Trombly, C. A., & Ma, H. (2002). A synthesis of the effects of occupational therapy for persons with stroke, part I: Restoration of roles, tasks, and activities. *American Journal of Occupational Therapy, 56,* 250–259.

Tse, T. (2005). The environment and falls prevention: Do environmental modifications make a difference? *Australian Occupational Therapy Journal, 52,* 271–281.

Health and Wellness

Case-Control and Cohort Designs

Classen, S., Mann, W., Wu, S. S., & Tomita, M. R. (2004). Relationship of number of medications to functional status, health, and quality of life for the frail home-based older adult. *OTJR: Occupation, Participation, and Health, 24,* 151–160.

Multiple-Treatment Designs

Lee, H. L., Tan, H. K.-L., Ma, H.-I., Tsai, C.-Y., & Liu, Y.-K. (2006). Effectiveness of a work-related stress management program in patients with chronic schizophrenia. *American Journal of Occupational Therapy, 60,* 435–441.

Rebeiro, K. L., Day, D. G., Semeniuk, B., O'Brien, M. C., & Wilson, B. (2001). Northern Initiative for Social Action: An occupation-based mental health program. *American Journal of Occupational Therapy, 55,* 493–500.

Reynolds, F. (2004). Textile art promoting well-being in long-term illness: Some general and specific influences. *Journal of Occupational Science, 11,* 58–67.

Outcomes Research

Frank, G., Fishman, M., Crowley, C., Blair, B., Murphy, S. T., Montoya, J. A., et al. (2001). The New Stories/New Cultures after-school enrichment program: A direct cultural intervention. *American Journal of Occupational Therapy, 55,* 501–508.

Hart, D. L., Tepper, S., & Lieberman, D. (2001). Changes in health status for persons with wrist or hand impairments receiving occupational therapy or physical therapy. *American Journal of Occupational Therapy, 55,* 68–74.

Guthrie, P. F., Westphal, L., Dahlman, B., Berg, M., Behnam, K., & Ferrell, D. (2004). A patient lifting intervention for preventing the work-related injuries of nurses. *Work, 22,* 79–88.

Lamb, A. L., Finlayson, M., Mathiowetz, V., & Chen, H. Y. (2005). The outcomes of using self-study modules in energy conservation education for people with multiple sclerosis. *Clinical Rehabilitation, 19,* 475–481.

Qualitative Research Designs

Chan, S. C. C. (2004). Chronic obstructive pulmonary disease and engagement in occupation. *American Journal of Occupational Therapy, 58,* 408–415.

Randomized Designs

Ivanoff, D., Sonn, S., & Svensson, E. (2002). A health education program for elderly persons with visual impairments and perceived security in the performance of daily occupations: A randomized study. *American Journal of Occupational Therapy, 56,* 322–330.

Mathiowetz, V., Finlayson, M. L., Matuska, K. M., Chen, H. Y., & Luo, P. (2005). Randomized control trial of an energy conservation course for persons with multiple sclerosis. *Multiple Sclerosis, 11,* 592–601.

Single-Case Research Designs

Holm, M. B., Santangelo, M. A., Fromuth, D. J., Brown, S. O., & Walter, H. (2000). Effectiveness of everyday occupations for changing client behaviors in a community living arrangement. *American Journal of Occupational Therapy, 54,* 361–371.

Systematic Evidence Reviews

Dinh-Zarr, T., Goss, C., Heitman, E., Roberts, I., & DiGuiseppi, C. (2004). Interventions for preventing injuries in problem drinkers. *Cochrane Database of Systematic Reviews,* Issue 3, CD001857. DOI:10.1002/14651858.CD001857.pub2.

Gillespie, L. D., Gillespie, W. J., Robertson, M. C., Lamb, S. E., Cumming, R. G., & Rowe, B. H. (2003). Interventions for preventing falls in elderly people. *Cochrane Database of Systematic Reviews,* Issue 4, CD000340. DOI:10.1002/14651858.CD000340.

Pekkala, E., & Merinder, L. (2002). Psychoeducation for schizophrenia. *Cochrane Database of Systematic Reviews,* Issue 2, CD002831. DOI:10.1002/14651858.CD002831.

Quality of Life

Case-Control and Cohort Designs

Classen, S., Mann, W., Wu, S. S., & Tomita, M. R. (2004). Relationship of number of medications to functional status, health, and quality of life for the frail home-based older adult. *OTJR: Occupation, Participation, and Health, 24,* 151–160.

Case Studies

Migliore, A. (2004). Improving dyspnea management in three adults with chronic obstructive pulmonary disease. *American Journal of Occupational Therapy, 58,* 639–646.

Outcomes Research

Case-Smith, J. (2003). Outcomes in hand rehabilitation using occupational therapy services. *American Journal of Occupational Therapy, 57,* 499–506.

Huebner, R. A., Johnson, K., Bennett, C. M., & Schneck, C. (2003). Community participation and quality of life outcomes after adult traumatic brain injury. *American Journal of Occupational Therapy, 57,* 177–185.

Qualitative Research Designs

Mathiowetz, V., Finlayson, M. L., Matuska, K. M., Chen, H. Y., & Luo, P. (2005). Randomized control trial of an energy conservation course for persons with multiple sclerosis. *Multiple Sclerosis, 11,* 592–601.

Rebeiro, K. L., Day, D. G., Semeniuk, B., O'Brien, M. C., & Wilson, B. (2001). Northern Initiative for Social Action: An occupation-based mental health program. *American Journal of Occupational Therapy, 55,* 493–500.

Reynolds, F. (2004). Textile art promoting well-being in long-term illness: Some general and specific influences. *Journal of Occupational Science, 11,* 58–67.

Siporin, S., & Lysack, C. (2004). Quality of life and supported employment: A case study of three women with developmental disabilities. *American Journal of Occupational Therapy, 58,* 455–465.

Randomized Designs

Dooley, N. R., & Hinojosa, J. (2004). Improving quality of life for persons with Alzheimer's disease and their family caregivers: Brief occupational therapy intervention. *American Journal of Occupational Therapy, 58,* 561–569.

Norweg, A. M., Whiteson, J., Malgady, R., Mola, A., & Rey, M. (2005). The effectiveness of different combinations of pulmonary rehabilitation program components: A randomized control trial. *Chest, 128,* 663–672.

Studenski, S., Duncan, P., Perera, S., Reker, D., Min Lai, S., & Richards, L. (2005). Daily functioning and quality of life in a randomized control trial of therapeutic exercise for subacute stroke survivors. *Stroke, 36,* 1764–1770.

Principles of Occupations Used for Intervention

1. Occupations and activities act as the therapeutic change agent to *remediate* and *restore*.

Case Studies

Earley, D., & Shannon, M. (2006). The use of occupation-based treatment with a person who has shoulder adhesive capsulitis: A case report. *American Journal of Occupational Therapy, 60,* 397–403.

Hurst, C. M. F., Van de Weyer, S., Smith, C., & Adler, P. M. (2006). Improvements in performance following optometric vision therapy in a child following dyspraxia. *Ophthalmic and Physiological Optics, 26,* 199–210.

Nilsson, L. M., & Nyberg, P. J. (2003). Driving to learn: A new concept for training children with profound cognitive disabilities in a powered wheelchair. *American Journal of Occupational Therapy, 57,* 229–233.

Phillips, M. E., Katz, J. A., & Harden, R. N. (2000). The use of nerve blocks in conjunction with occupational therapy for complex regional pain syndrome type I. *American Journal of Occupational Therapy, 54,* 544–549.

Meta-analyses

Murphy, S., & Tickle-Degnen, L. (2001). The effectiveness of occupational therapy related treatments for persons with Parkinson's disease: A meta-analytic review. *American Journal of Occupational Therapy, 55,* 385–392.

Walker, M. F., Leonardi-Bee, J., Bath, P., Landhorne, P., Dewey, M., Corr, S., et al. (2004). Individual patient data meta-analysis of randomized control trials of community occupational therapy for stroke patients. *Stroke, 35,* 2226–2232.

Nonrandomized Designs

Case-Smith, J. (2002). Effectiveness of school-based occupational therapy intervention on handwriting. *American Journal of Occupational Therapy, 56,* 17–25.

Jackson, J. P., & Schkade, J. K. (2001). Occupational adaptation model versus biomechanical–rehabilitation model in the treatment of patients with hip fractures. *American Journal of Occupational Therapy, 55,* 531–537.

Landi, F., Cesari, M., Onder, G., Tafani, A., Zamboni, V., & Cocchi, A. (2006). Effects of an occupational therapy program on functional outcomes in older stroke patients. *Gerontology, 52,* 85–91.

Smith, S. A., Press, B., Koenig, K. P., & Kinnealey, M. (2005). Effects of sensory integration intervention on self-stimulating and self-injurious behaviors. *American Journal of Occupational Therapy, 59,* 418–425.

Outcomes Research

Case-Smith, J. (2003). Outcomes in hand rehabilitation using occupational therapy services. *American Journal of Occupational Therapy, 57,* 499–506.

Dankert, H. L., Davies, P. L., & Gavin, W. L. (2003). Occupational therapy effects on visual–motor skills in preschool children. *American Journal of Occupational Therapy, 57,* 542–549.

Lavelle, P., & Tomlin, G. S. (2001). Occupational therapy goal achievement for persons with postacute cerebrovascular accident in an on-campus student clinic. *American Journal of Occupational Therapy, 55,* 36–42.

Lysack, C. L., MacNeill, S. E., & Lichtenberg, P. A. (2001). The functional performance of elderly urban African-American women who return home to live alone after medical rehabilitation. *American Journal of Occupational Therapy, 55,* 433–440.

Marr, D., & Dimeo, S. B. (2006). Outcomes associated with a summer handwriting course for elementary students. *American Journal of Occupational Therapy, 60,* 10–15.

Sharek, P. J., Wayman, K., Lin, E., Strichartz, D., Sentivany-Collins, S., Good, J., et al. (2006). Improved pain management in pediatric postoperative liver transplant patients using parental education and non-pharmacological interventions. *Pediatric Transplantation, 10,* 172–177.

Qualitative Research Designs

Gillot, A. J., Holder-Walls, A., Kurtz, J. R., & Varley, N. C. (2003). Perceptions and experiences of two survivors of stroke who participated in constraint-induced movement therapy home programs. *American Journal of Occupational Therapy, 57,* 139–151.

Randomized Designs

Cheng, A. S.-K. (2000). Use of early tactile stimulation in rehabilitation of digital nerve injuries. *American Journal of Occupational Therapy, 54,* 159–165.

Norweg, A. M., Whiteson, J., Malgady, R., Mola, A., & Rey, M. (2005). The effectiveness of different combinations of pulmonary rehabilitation program components: A randomized control trial. *Chest, 128,* 663–672.

Peterson, C. Q., & Nelson, D. L. (2003). Effect of an occupational intervention on printing in children with economic disadvantages. *American Journal of Occupational Therapy, 57,* 152–160.

Shaffer, R. J., Jacokes, L. E., Cassily, J. F., Greenspan, S. I., Tuchman, R. F., & Temmer, P. J., Jr. (2001). Effect of interactive Metronome® training on children with ADHD. *American Journal of Occupational Therapy, 55,* 155–162.

Sung, I., Ryu, J., Pyun, S., Yoo, S., Song, W., & Park, M. (2005). Efficacy of forced-use therapy in hemiplegic cerebral palsy. *Archives of Physical Medicine Rehabilitation, 86,* 2195–2198.

Single-Case Research Designs

Deitz, J., Swinth, Y., & White, O. (2002). Powered mobility and preschoolers with complex developmental delays. *American Journal of Occupational Therapy, 56,* 86–96.

Hällgren, M., & Kottorp, A. (2005). Effects of occupational therapy intervention on activities of daily living and awareness of disability in persons with intellectual disabilities. *Australian Occupational Therapy Journal, 52,* 350–359.

Handley-More, D., Deitz, J., Billingsley, F. F., & Coggins, T. E. (2003). Facilitating written work using computer word processing and word prediction. *American Journal of Occupational Therapy, 57,* 139–151.

Melchert-McKearnan, K., Deitz, J., Engel, J. M., & White, O. (2000). Children with burn injuries: Purposeful activity versus rote exercise. *American Journal of Occupational Therapy, 54,* 381–390.

Tham, K., Ginsburg, E., Fisher, A. G., & Tegnér, R. (2001). Training to improve awareness of disabilities in clients with unilateral neglect. *American Journal of Occupational Therapy, 55,* 46–54.

Systematic Reviews

Guzmán, J., Esmail, R., Karjalainen, K., Malmivaara, A., Irvin, E., & Bombardier, C. (2002). Multidisciplinary bio-psycho-social rehabilitation for chronic low-back pain. *Cochrane Database of Systematic Reviews,* Issue 1, CD000963. DOI: 10.1002/14651858.CD000963.

Schonstein, E., Kenny, D. T., Keating, J., & Koes, B. W. (2003). Work conditioning, work hardening, and functional restoration for workers with back and neck pain. *Cochrane Database of Systematic Reviews,* Issue 3, CD001822. DOI:10.1002/14651858.CD001822.

Steultjens, E. E. M. J., Bouter, L. L. M., Dekker, J. J., Kuyk, M. M. A. H., Schaardenberg, D. D., & Van den Ende, E. C. H. M. (2004). Occupational therapy for rheumatoid arthritis. *Cochrane Database of Systematic Reviews,* Issue 1, CD003114. DOI: 10.1002/14651858.CD003114.pub2.

Stoffel, V. C., & Moyers, P. A. (2004). An evidence-based and occupational perspective of interventions for persons with substance-use disorders. *American Journal of Occupational Therapy, 56,* 570–586.

Trombly, C. A., & Ma, H. (2002). A synthesis of the effects of occupational therapy for persons with stroke, part I: Restoration of roles, tasks, and activities. *American Journal of Occupational Therapy, 56,* 250–259.

Woods, B., Spector, A., Jones, C., Orrell, M., & Davies, S. (2005). Reminiscence therapy for dementia. *Cochrane Database of Systematic Reviews,* Issue 2, CD001120. DOI:10.1002/14651858.CD001120.pub2.

2. The use of new occupations as interventions provides the means for *establishing* performance skills and for developing habits.

Case Studies

Legault, E., & Rebeiro, K. L. (2001). Occupation as means to mental health: A single case study. *American Journal of Occupational Therapy, 55,* 90–96.

Meta-analyses

Murphy, S., & Tickle-Degnen, L. (2001). The effectiveness of occupational therapy–related treatments for persons with Parkinson's disease: A meta-analytic review. *American Journal of Occupational Therapy, 55,* 385–392.

Walker, M. F., Leonardi-Bee, J., Bath, P., Landhorne, P., Dewey, M., Corr, S., et al. (2004). Individual patient data meta-analysis of randomized control trials of community occupational therapy for stroke patients. *Stroke, 35,* 2226–2232.

Nonrandomized Designs

Case-Smith, J. (2002). Effectiveness of school-based occupational therapy intervention on handwriting. *American Journal of Occupational Therapy, 56,* 17–25.

Dankert, H. L., Davies, P. L., & Gavin, W. L. (2003). Occupational therapy effects on visual–motor skills in preschool children. *American Journal of Occupational Therapy, 57,* 542–549.

Dreiling, D. S., & Bundy, A. C. (2003). A comparison of consultative model and direct–indirect intervention with preschoolers. *American Journal of Occupational Therapy, 57,* 566–569.

Jackson, J. P., & Schkade, J. K. (2001). Occupational adaptation model versus biomechanical–rehabilitation model in the treatment of patients with hip fractures. *American Journal of Occupational Therapy, 55,* 531–537.

Landi, F., Cesari, M., Onder, G., Tafani, A., Zamboni, V., & Cocchi, A. (2006). Effects of an occupational therapy program on functional outcomes in older stroke patients. *Gerontology, 52,* 85–91.

Outcomes Research

Frank, G., Fishman, M., Crowley, C., Blair, B., Murphy, S. T., Montoya, J. A., et al. (2001). The New Stories/New Cultures after-school enrichment program: A direct cultural intervention. *American Journal of Occupational Therapy, 55,* 501–508.

Lysack, C. L., MacNeill, S. E., & Lichtenberg, P. A. (2001). The functional performance of elderly urban African-American women who return home to live alone after medical rehabilitation. *American Journal of Occupational Therapy, 55,* 433–440.

Marr, D., & Dimeo, S. B. (2006). Outcomes associated with a summer handwriting course for elementary students. *American Journal of Occupational Therapy, 60,* 10–15.

Qualitative Research Designs

Camp, M. M. (2001). The use of service dogs as an adaptive strategy: A qualitative study. *American Journal of Occupational Therapy, 55,* 509–517.

Copolillo, A., & Teitelman, J. L. (2005). Acquisition and integration of low vision assistive devices: Understanding the decision-making process of older adults with low vision. *American Journal of Occupational Therapy, 59,* 305–313.

Howie, L., Coulter, M., & Feldman, S. (2004). Crafting the self: Older persons' narratives of occupational identity. *American Journal of Occupational Therapy, 58,* 446–454.

Kielhofner, G., Braveman, B., Finlayson, M., Paul-Ward, A., Goldbaum, L., & Goldstein, K. (2004). Outcomes of a vocation program for persons with AIDS. *American Journal of Occupational Therapy, 58,* 64–72.

Rebeiro, K. L., Day, D. G., Semeniuk, B., O'Brien, M. C., & Wilson, B. (2001). Northern Initiative for Social Action: An occupation-based mental health program. *American Journal of Occupational Therapy, 55,* 493–500.

Randomized Designs

Peterson, C. Q., & Nelson, D. L. (2003). Effect of an occupational intervention on printing in children with economic disadvantages. *American Journal of Occupational Therapy, 57,* 152–160.

Sung, I., Ryu, J., Pyun, S., Yoo, S., Song, W., & Park, M. (2005). Efficacy of forced-use therapy in hemiplegic cerebral palsy. *Archives of Physical Medicine Rehabilitation, 86,* 2195–2198.

Single-Case Research Designs

Hällgren, M., & Kottorp, A. (2005). Effects of occupational therapy intervention on activities of daily living and awareness of disability in persons with intellectual disabilities. *Australian Occupational Therapy Journal, 52,* 350–359.

Handley-More, D., Deitz, J., Billingsley, F. F., & Coggins, T. E. (2003). Facilitating written work using computer word processing and word prediction. *American Journal of Occupational Therapy, 57,* 139–151.

Labelle, K.-L., & Mihaildis, A. (2006). The use of automated prompting to facilitate handwashing in persons with dementia. *American Journal of Occupational Therapy, 60,* 442–450.

Tham, K., Ginsburg, E., Fisher, A. G., & Tegnér, R. (2001). Training to improve awareness of disabilities in clients with unilateral neglect. *American Journal of Occupational Therapy, 55,* 46–54.

Systematic Reviews

Outpatient Service Trialists. (2003). Therapy-based rehabilitation services for stroke patients at home. *Cochrane Database of Systematic Reviews,* Issue 1, CD002925. DOI:10.1002/14651858. CD002925.

Stoffel, V. C., & Moyers, P. A. (2004). An evidence-based and occupational perspective of interventions for persons with substance-use disorders. *American Journal of Occupational Therapy, 56,* 570–586.

Trombly, C. A., & Ma, H. (2002). A synthesis of the effects of occupational therapy for persons with stroke, part I: Restoration of roles, tasks, and activities. *American Journal of Occupational Therapy, 56,* 250–259.

Turner-Stokes, L., Disler, P. B., Nair, A., & Wade, D. T. (2005). Multi-disciplinary rehabilitation for acquired brain injury in adults of working age. *Cochrane Database of Systematic Reviews,* Issue 3, CD004170. DOI:10.1002/14651858.CD004170. pub2.

3. Valued occupations are *inherently motivating.*

Nonrandomized Designs

Jackson, J. P., & Schkade, J. K. (2001). Occupational adaptation model versus biomechanical–rehabilitation model in the treatment of patients with hip fractures. *American Journal of Occupational Therapy, 55,* 531–537.

Qualitative Research Designs

Chan, J., & Spencer, J. (2004). Adaptation to hand injury: An evolving experience. *American Journal of Occupational Therapy, 58,* 128–139.

Gillot, A. J., Holder-Walls, A., Kurtz, J. R., & Varley, N. C. (2003). Perceptions and experiences of two survivors of stroke who participated in constraint-induced movement therapy home programs. *American Journal of Occupational Therapy, 57,* 139–151.

Rebeiro, K. L., Day, D. G., Semeniuk, B., O'Brien, M. C., & Wilson, B. (2001). Northern Initiative for Social Action: An occupation-based mental health program. *American Journal of Occupational Therapy, 55,* 493–500.

Siporin, S., & Lysack, C. (2004). Quality of life and supported employment: A case study of three women with developmental disabilities. *American Journal of Occupational Therapy, 58,* 455–465.

Single-Case Research Designs

Deitz, J., Swinth, Y., & White, O. (2002). Powered mobility and preschoolers with complex developmental delays. *American Journal of Occupational Therapy, 56,* 86–96.

Melchert-McKearnan, K., Deitz, J., Engel, J. M., & White, O. (2000). Children with burn injuries: Purposeful activity versus rote exercise. *American Journal of Occupational Therapy, 54,* 381–390.

Tham, K., Ginsburg, E., Fisher, A. G., & Tegnér, R. (2001). Training to improve awareness of disabilities in clients with unilateral neglect. *American Journal of Occupational Therapy, 55,* 46–54.

4. Occupations promote the identification of *values* and *interests*.

Outcomes Research

Frank, G., Fishman, M., Crowley, C., Blair, B., Murphy, S. T., Montoya, J. A., et al. (2001). The New Stories/New Cultures after-school enrichment program: A direct cultural intervention. *American Journal of Occupational Therapy, 55,* 501–508.

Qualitative Research Designs

Chan, S. C. C. (2004). Chronic obstructive pulmonary disease and engagement in occupation. *American Journal of Occupational Therapy, 58,* 408–415.

Howie, L., Coulter, M., & Feldman, S. (2004). Crafting the self: Older persons' narratives of occupational identity. *American Journal of Occupational Therapy, 58,* 446–454.

Rebeiro, K. L., Day, D. G., Semeniuk, B., O'Brien, M. C., & Wilson, B. (2001). Northern Initiative for Social Action: An occupation-based mental health program. *American Journal of Occupational Therapy, 55,* 493–500.

Siporin, S., & Lysack, C. (2004). Quality of life and supported employment: A case study of three women with developmental disabilities. *American Journal of Occupational Therapy, 58,* 455–465.

Spencer, J., Hersch, G., Shelton, M., Ripple, J., Spencer, C., Dyer, C. B., et al. (2002). Functional outcomes and daily life activities of African-American elders after hospitalization. *American Journal of Occupational Therapy, 56,* 149–159.

Randomized Designs

Jarus, T., Shavit, S., & Ratzon, N. (2000). From hand twister to mind twister: Computer-aided treatment in traumatic wrist fracture. *American Journal of Occupational Therapy, 54,* 176–182.

Single-Case Research Designs

Tham, K., Ginsburg, E., Fisher, A. G., & Tegnér, R. (2001). Training to improve awareness of disabilities in clients with unilateral neglect. *American Journal of Occupational Therapy, 55,* 46–54.

5. Occupations create opportunities to *practice* performance skills and to *reinforce* performance.

Case Studies

Legault, E., & Rebeiro, K. L. (2001). Occupation as means to mental health: A single case study. *American Journal of Occupational Therapy, 55,* 90–96.

Nonrandomized Designs

Jackson, J. P., & Schkade, J. K. (2001). Occupational adaptation model versus biomechanical–rehabilitation model in the treatment of patients with hip fractures. *American Journal of Occupational Therapy, 55,* 531–537.

Landi, F., Cesari, M., Onder, G., Tafani, A., Zamboni, V., & Cocchi, A. (2006). Effects of an occupational therapy program on functional outcomes in older stroke patients. *Gerontology, 52,* 85–91.

Outcomes Research

Frank, G., Fishman, M., Crowley, C., Blair, B., Murphy, S. T., Montoya, J. A., et al. (2001). The New Stories/New Cultures after-school enrichment program: A direct cultural intervention. *American Journal of Occupational Therapy, 55,* 501–508.

Lysack, C. L., MacNeill, S. E., & Lichtenberg, P. A. (2001). The functional performance of elderly urban African-American women who return home to live alone after medical rehabilitation. *American Journal of Occupational Therapy, 55,* 433–440.

Marr, D., & Dimeo, S. B. (2006). Outcomes associated with a summer handwriting course for elementary students. *American Journal of Occupational Therapy, 60,* 10–15.

Oka, M., Otsuka, K., Yokoyama, N., Mintz, J., Hoshino, K., Niwa, S.-I., et al. (2004). An evaluation of a hybrid occupational therapy supported employment program in Japan for persons with schizophrenia. *American Journal of Occupational Therapy, 58,* 466–475.

Qualitative Research Designs

Camp, M. M. (2001). The use of service dogs as an adaptive strategy: A qualitative study. *American Journal of Occupational Therapy, 55,* 509–517.

Dale, L. (2004). Partnering with management to implement ergonomics in the industrial setting. *Work, 22,* 117–124.

Gillot, A. J., Holder-Walls, A., Kurtz, J. R., & Varley, N. C. (2003). Perceptions and experiences of two survivors of stroke who participated in constraint-induced movement therapy home programs. *American Journal of Occupational Therapy, 57,* 139–151.

Howie, L., Coulter, M., & Feldman, S. (2004). Crafting the self: Older persons' narratives of occupational identity. *American Journal of Occupational Therapy, 58,* 446–454.

Rebeiro, K. L., Day, D. G., Semeniuk, B., O'Brien, M. C., & Wilson, B. (2001). Northern Initiative for Social Action: An occupation-based mental health program. *American Journal of Occupational Therapy, 55,* 493–500.

Randomized Designs

Jarus, T., Shavit, S., & Ratzon, N. (2000). From hand twister to mind twister: Computer-aided treatment in traumatic wrist fracture. *American Journal of Occupational Therapy, 54,* 176–182.

Peterson, C. Q., & Nelson, D. L. (2003). Effect of an occupational intervention on printing in children with economic disadvantages. *American Journal of Occupational Therapy, 57,* 152–160.

Sung, I., Ryu, J., Pyun, S., Yoo, S., Song, W., & Park, M. (2005). Efficacy of forced-use therapy in hemiplegic cerebral palsy. *Archives of Physical Medicine Rehabilitation, 86,* 2195–2198.

Single-Case Research Designs

Hällgren, M., & Kottorp, A. (2005). Effects of occupational therapy intervention on activities of daily living and awareness of disability in persons with intellectual disabilities. *Australian Occupational Therapy Journal, 52,* 350–359.

Tham, K., Ginsburg, E., Fisher, A. G., & Tegnér, R. (2001). Training to improve awareness of disabilities in clients with unilateral neglect. *American Journal of Occupational Therapy, 55,* 46–54.

Systematic Reviews

Outpatient Service Trialists. (2003). Therapy-based rehabilitation services for stroke patients at home. *Cochrane Database of Systematic Reviews,* Issue 1, CD002925. DOI:10.1002/14651858. CD002925.

Trombly, C. A., & Ma, H. (2002). A synthesis of the effects of occupational therapy for persons with stroke, part I: Restoration of roles, tasks, and activities. *American Journal of Occupational Therapy, 56,* 250–259.

Turner-Stokes, L., Disler, P. B., Nair, A., & Wade, D. T. (2005). Multi-disciplinary rehabilitation for acquired brain injury in adults of working age. *Cochrane Database of Systematic Reviews,* Issue 3, CD004170. DOI:10.1002/14651858.CD004170. pub2.

6. Active engagement in occupations produces *feedback*.

Nonrandomized Designs

Dankert, H. L., Davies, P. L., & Gavin, W. L. (2003). Occupational therapy effects on visual–motor skills in preschool children. *American Journal of Occupational Therapy, 57,* 542–549.

Randomized Designs

Jarus, T., Shavit, S., & Ratzon, N. (2000). From hand twister to mind twister: Computer-aided treatment in traumatic wrist fracture. *American Journal of Occupational Therapy, 54,* 176–182.

Peterson, C. Q., & Nelson, D. L. (2003). Effect of an occupational intervention on printing in children with economic disadvantages. *American Journal of Occupational Therapy, 57,* 152–160.

Shaffer, R. J., Jacokes, L. E., Cassily, J. F., Greenspan, S. I., Tuchman, R. F., & Temmer, P. J., Jr. (2001). Effect of interactive Metronome® training on children with ADHD. *American Journal of Occupational Therapy, 55,* 155–162.

Sung, I., Ryu, J., Pyun, S., Yoo, S., Song, W., & Park, M. (2005). Efficacy of forced-use therapy in hemiplegic cerebral palsy. *Archives of Physical Medicine Rehabilitation, 86,* 2195–2198.

Qualitative Research Designs

Gillot, A. J., Holder-Walls, A., Kurtz, J. R., & Varley, N. C. (2003). Perceptions and experiences of two survivors of stroke who participated in constraint-induced movement therapy home programs. *American Journal of Occupational Therapy, 57,* 139–151.

Single-Case Research Designs

Deitz, J., Swinth, Y., & White, O. (2002). Powered mobility and preschoolers with complex developmental delays. *American Journal of Occupational Therapy, 56,* 86–96.

Labelle, K.-L., & Mihaildis, A. (2006). The use of automated prompting to facilitate handwashing in persons with dementia. *American Journal of Occupational Therapy, 60,* 442–450.

Schilling, D. L., Washington, K., Billingsley, F. F., & Deitz, J. (2003). Classroom seating for children with attention deficit hyperactivity disorder: Therapy balls versus chairs. *American Journal of Occupational Therapy, 57,* 534–541.

Tham, K., Ginsburg, E., Fisher, A. G., & Tegnér, R. (2001). Training to improve awareness of disabilities in clients with unilateral neglect. *American Journal of Occupational Therapy, 55,* 46–54.

Systematic Reviews

Trombly, C. A., & Ma, H. (2002). A synthesis of the effects of occupational therapy for persons with stroke, part I: Restoration of roles, tasks, and activities. *American Journal of Occupational Therapy, 56,* 250–259.

7. Engagement in occupations facilitates *mastery* or *competence* in performing daily activities.

Case-Control and Cohort Designs

MacKinnon, J. R., & Miller, W. C. (2003). Rheumatoid arthritis and self-esteem: The impact of quality occupation. *Journal of Occupational Science, 10,* 90–98.

Schmidt Hanson, C., Nabavi, D., & Yuen, H. K. (2001). The effect of sports on level of commu-

nity integration as reported by persons with spinal cord injury. *American Journal of Occupational Therapy, 55,* 332–338.

Meta-Analyses

Walker, M. F., Leonardi-Bee, J., Bath, P., Landhorne, P., Dewey, M., Corr, S., et al. (2004). Individual patient data meta-analysis of randomized control trials of community occupational therapy for stroke patients. *Stroke, 35,* 2226–2232.

Nonrandomized Designs

Fasoli, S. E., Trombly, C. A., Tickle-Degnen, L., & Verfaellie, M. H. (2002). Effect of instruction on functional reach in persons with and without cerebrovascular accident. *American Journal of Occupational Therapy, 56,* 380–390.

Landi, F., Cesari, M., Onder, G., Tafani, A., Zamboni, V., & Cocchi, A. (2006). Effects of an occupational therapy program on functional outcomes in older stroke patients. *Gerontology, 52,* 85–91.

Qualitative Research Designs

Camp, M. M. (2001). The use of service dogs as an adaptive strategy: A qualitative study. *American Journal of Occupational Therapy, 55,* 509–517.

Ganstrom-Strandqvist, K., Liukko, A., & Tham, K. (2003). The meaning of the working cooperative for persons with long-term mental illness: A phenomenological study. *American Journal of Occupational Therapy, 57,* 262–272.

Gillot, A. J., Holder-Walls, A., Kurtz, J. R., & Varley, N. C. (2003). Perceptions and experiences of two survivors of stroke who participated in constraint-induced movement therapy home programs. *American Journal of Occupational Therapy, 57,* 139–151.

Howie, L., Coulter, M., & Feldman, S. (2004). Crafting the self: Older persons' narratives of occupational identity. *American Journal of Occupational Therapy, 58,* 446–454.

Rebeiro, K. L., Day, D. G., Semeniuk, B., O'Brien, M. C., & Wilson, B. (2001). Northern Initiative for Social Action: An occupation-based mental health program. *American Journal of Occupational Therapy, 55,* 493–500.

Randomized Designs

Peterson, C. Q., & Nelson, D. L. (2003). Effect of an occupational intervention on printing in children with economic disadvantages. *American Journal of Occupational Therapy, 57,* 152–160.

Single-Case Research Designs

Deitz, J., Swinth, Y., & White, O. (2002). Powered mobility and preschoolers with complex developmental delays. *American Journal of Occupational Therapy, 56,* 86–96.

8. Selected occupations promote *participation* with persons or groups.

Case-Control and Cohort Designs

Schmidt Hanson, C., Nabavi, D., & Yuen, H. K. (2001). The effect of sports on level of community integration as reported by persons with spinal cord injury. *American Journal of Occupational Therapy, 55,* 332–338.

Case Studies

Legault, E., & Rebeiro, K. L. (2001). Occupation as means to mental health: A single case study. *American Journal of Occupational Therapy, 55,* 90–96.

Nonrandomized Designs

Trombly, C. A., Radomski, M. V., Trexel, C., & Burnett-Smith, S. E. (2002). Occupational therapy and achievement of self-identified goals by adults with acquired brain injury: Phase II. *American Journal of Occupational Therapy, 56,* 489–498.

Outcomes Research

Camp, M. M. (2001). The use of service dogs as an adaptive strategy: A qualitative study. *American Journal of Occupational Therapy, 55,* 509–517.

Case-Smith, J. (2003). Outcomes in hand rehabilitation using occupational therapy services. *American Journal of Occupational Therapy, 57,* 499–506.

Chan, S. C. C. (2004). Chronic obstructive pulmonary disease and engagement in occupation. *American Journal of Occupational Therapy, 58,* 408–415.

Huebner, R. A., Johnson, K., Bennett, C. M., & Schneck, C. (2003). Community participation

and quality of life outcomes after adult traumatic brain injury. *American Journal of Occupational Therapy, 57,* 177–185.

Oka, M., Otsuka, K., Yokoyama, N., Mintz, J., Hoshino, K., Niwa, S.-I., et al. (2004). An evaluation of a hybrid occupational therapy supported employment program in Japan for persons with schizophrenia. *American Journal of Occupational Therapy, 58,* 466–475.

Rebeiro, K. L., Day, D. G., Semeniuk, B., O'Brien, M. C., & Wilson, B. (2001). Northern Initiative for Social Action: An occupation-based mental health program. *American Journal of Occupational Therapy, 55,* 493–500.

Qualitative Research Designs

Camp, M. M. (2001). The use of service dogs as an adaptive strategy: A qualitative study. *American Journal of Occupational Therapy, 55,* 509–517.

Chan, J., & Spencer, J. (2004). Adaptation to hand injury: An evolving experience. *American Journal of Occupational Therapy, 58,* 128–139.

Howie, L., Coulter, M., & Feldman, S. (2004). Crafting the self: Older persons' narratives of occupational identity. *American Journal of Occupational Therapy, 58,* 446–454.

Rebeiro, K. L., Day, D. G., Semeniuk, B., O'Brien, M. C., & Wilson, B. (2001). Northern Initiative for Social Action: An occupation-based mental health program. *American Journal of Occupational Therapy, 55,* 493–500.

Spencer, J., Hersch, G., Shelton, M., Ripple, J., Spencer, C., Dyer, C. B., et al. (2002). Functional outcomes and daily life activities of African-American elders after hospitalization. *American Journal of Occupational Therapy, 56,* 149–159.

Single-Case Research Designs

Deitz, J., Swinth, Y., & White, O. (2002). Powered mobility and preschoolers with complex developmental delays. *American Journal of Occupational Therapy, 56,* 86–96.

Holm, M. B., Santangelo, M. A., Fromuth, D. J., Brown, S. O., & Walter, H. (2000). Effectiveness of everyday occupations for changing client behaviors in a community living arrangement.

American Journal of Occupational Therapy, 54, 361–371.

Tanta, K. J., Deitz, J. C., White, O., & Billingsley, F. (2005). The effects of peer-play level on initiations and responses of preschool children with delayed play skills. *American Journal of Occupational Therapy, 59,* 437–445.

Systematic Reviews

Han, A., Judd, M. G., Robinson, V. A., Taixiang, W., Tugwell, P., & Wells, G. (2004). Tai chi for treating rheumatoid arthritis. *Cochrane Database of Systematic Reviews,* Issue 3, CD004849. DOI: 10.1002/14651858.CD004849.

Stoffel, V. C., & Moyers, P. A. (2004). An evidence-based and occupational perspective of interventions for persons with substance-use disorders. *American Journal of Occupational Therapy, 56,* 570–586.

Trombly, C. A., & Ma, H. (2002). A synthesis of the effects of occupational therapy for persons with stroke, part I: Restoration of roles, tasks, and activities. *American Journal of Occupational Therapy, 56,* 250–259.

Woods, B., Spector, A., Jones, C., Orrell, M., & Davies, S. (2005). Reminiscence therapy for dementia. *Cochrane Database of Systematic Reviews,* Issue 2, CD001120. DOI:10.1002/ 14651858.CD001120.pub2.

9. Through engagement in occupations, persons learn to *assume responsibility for their own health and wellness.* Occupations exert a positive influence on *health* and *well-being* (Law, 2002b).

Outcomes Research

Frank, G., Fishman, M., Crowley, C., Blair, B., Murphy, S. T., Montoya, J. A., et al. (2001). The New Stories/New Cultures after-school enrichment program: A direct cultural intervention. *American Journal of Occupational Therapy, 55,* 501–508.

Lamb, A. L., Finlayson, M., Mathiowetz, V., & Chen, H. Y. (2005). The outcomes of using self-study modules in energy conservation education for people with multiple sclerosis. *Clinical Rehabilitation, 19,* 475–481.

Qualitative Research Designs

Chan, S. C. C. (2004). Chronic obstructive pulmonary disease and engagement in occupation. *American Journal of Occupational Therapy,, 58,* 408–415.

Rebeiro, K. L., Day, D. G., Semeniuk, B., O'Brien, M. C., & Wilson, B. (2001). Northern Initiative for Social Action: An occupation-based mental health program. *American Journal of Occupational Therapy, 55,* 493–500.

Reynolds, F. (2004). Textile art promoting well-being in long-term illness: Some general and specific influences. *Journal of Occupational Science, 11,* 58–67.

Randomized Designs

Ivanoff, D., Sonn, S., & Svensson, E. (2002). A health education program for elderly persons with visual impairments and perceived security in the performance of daily occupations: A randomized study. *American Journal of Occupational Therapy, 56,* 322–330.

Systematic Evidence Reviews

Gillespie L. D., Gillespie W. J., Robertson M. C., Lamb S. E., Cumming R. G., & Rowe B. H. (2003). Interventions for preventing falls in elderly people. *Cochrane Database of Systematic Reviews,* Issue 4, CD000340. DOI: 10.1002/14651858. CD000340.

Stoffel, V. C., & Moyers, P. A. (2004). An evidence-based and occupational perspective of interventions for persons with substance-use disorders. *American Journal of Occupational Therapy, 56,* 570–586.

10. Occupations provide the means for persons to *adapt* to changing needs and conditions.

Case Studies

Erhardt, R. P., & Meade, V. (2005). Improving handwriting without teaching handwriting: The consultative clinical reasoning process. *Australian Occupational Therapy Journal, 52,* 199–210.

Phillips, M. E., Katz, J. A., & Harden, R. N. (2000). The use of nerve blocks in conjunction with occupational therapy for complex regional pain syndrome type I. *American Journal of Occupational Therapy, 54,* 544–549.

Nonrandomized Designs

Dankert, H. L., Davies, P. L., & Gavin, W. L. (2003). Occupational therapy effects on visual–motor skills in preschool children. *American Journal of Occupational Therapy, 57,* 542–549.

Dreiling, D. S., & Bundy, A. C. (2003). A comparison of consultative model and direct–indirect intervention with preschoolers. *American Journal of Occupational Therapy, 57,* 566–569.

Fasoli, S. E., Trombly, C. A., Tickle-Degnen, L., & Verfaellie, M. H. (2002). Effect of instruction on functional reach in persons with and without cerebrovascular accident. *American Journal of Occupational Therapy, 56,* 380–390.

Jackson, J. P., & Schkade, J. K. (2001). Occupational adaptation model versus biomechanical–rehabilitation model in the treatment of patients with hip fractures. *American Journal of Occupational Therapy, 55,* 531–537.

Landi, F., Cesari, M., Onder, G., Tafani, A., Zamboni, V., & Cocchi, A. (2006). Effects of an occupational therapy program on functional outcomes in older stroke patients. *Gerontology, 52,* 85–91.

Trombly, C. A., Radomski, M. V., Trexel, C., & Burnett-Smith, S. E. (2002). Occupational therapy and achievement of self-identified goals by adults with acquired brain injury: Phase II. *American Journal of Occupational Therapy, 56,* 489–498.

Outcomes Research

Droeze, E. H., & Jonsson, H. (2005). Evaluation of ergonomic interventions to reduce musculoskeletal disorders of dentists in the Netherlands. *Work, 25,* 211–220.

Lysack, C. L., MacNeill, S. E., & Lichtenberg, P. A. (2001). The functional performance of elderly urban African-American women who return home to live alone after medical rehabilitation. *American Journal of Occupational Therapy, 55,* 433–440.

Qualitative Research Designs

Bontje, P., Kinébanian, A., Josephsson, S., & Tamura, Y. (2004). Occupational adaptation: The experiences of older persons with physical disabilities. *American Journal of Occupational Therapy, 58,* 140–149.

Camp, M. M. (2001). The use of service dogs as an adaptive strategy: A qualitative study. *American Journal of Occupational Therapy, 55,* 509–517.

Copolillo, A., & Teitelman, J. L. (2005). Acquisition and integration of low vision assistive devices: Understanding the decision-making process of older adults with low vision. *American Journal of Occupational Therapy, 59,* 305–313.

Erikson, A., Karlsson, G., Söderström, K., & Tham, K. (2004). A training apartment with electronic aids to daily living: Lived experiences of persons with brain damage. *American Journal of Occupational Therapy, 58,* 261–271.

Gillot, A. J., Holder-Walls, A., Kurtz, J. R., & Varley, N. C. (2003). Perceptions and experiences of two survivors of stroke who participated in constraint-induced movement therapy home programs. *American Journal of Occupational Therapy, 57,* 139–151.

Spencer, J., Hersch, G., Shelton, M., Ripple, J., Spencer, C., Dyer, C. B., et al. (2002). Functional outcomes and daily life activities of African-American elders after hospitalization. *American Journal of Occupational Therapy, 56,* 149–159.

Randomized Designs

Dooley, N. R., & Hinojosa, J. (2004). Improving quality of life for persons with Alzheimer's disease and their family caregivers: Brief occupational therapy intervention. *American Journal of Occupational Therapy, 58,* 561–569.

Mathiowetz, V., Finlayson, M. L., Matuska, K. M., Chen, H. Y., & Luo, P. (2005). Randomized control trial of an energy conservation course for persons with multiple sclerosis. *Multiple Sclerosis, 11,* 592–601.

Single-Case Research Designs

McGruder, J., Cors, D., Tiernan, A. M., & Tomlin, G. (2003). Weighted wrist cuffs for tremor reduction during eating in adults with static brain lesions. *American Journal of Occupational Therapy, 57*, 507–516.

Schilling, D. L., Washington, K., Billingsley, F. F., & Deitz, J. (2003). Classroom seating for children with attention deficit hyperactivity disorder: Therapy balls versus chairs. *American Journal of Occupational Therapy, 57*, 534–541.

Tham, K., Ginsburg, E., Fisher, A. G., & Tegnér, R. (2001). Training to improve awareness of disabilities in clients with unilateral neglect. *American Journal of Occupational Therapy, 55*, 46–54.

Systematic Reviews

Gillespie, L. D., Gillespie, W. J., Robertson, M. C., Lamb, S. E., Cumming, R. G., & Rowe, B. H. (2003). Interventions for preventing falls in elderly people. *Cochrane Database of Systematic Reviews,* Issue 4, CD000340. DOI:10.1002/14651858.CD000340.

Trombly, C. A., & Ma, H. (2002). A synthesis of the effects of occupational therapy for persons with stroke, part I: Restoration of roles, tasks, and activities. *American Journal of Occupational Therapy, 56*, 250–259.

Tse, T. (2005). The environment and falls prevention: Do environmental modifications make a difference? *Australian Occupational Therapy Journal, 52*, 271–281.

11. Occupations contribute to the creation and maintenance of *identity* (AOTA, 2002; Christiansen, 1999).

Qualitative Research Designs

Chan, S. C. C. (2004). Chronic obstructive pulmonary disease and engagement in occupation. *American Journal of Occupational Therapy, 58*, 408–415.

Howie, L., Coulter, M., & Feldman, S. (2004). Crafting the self: Older persons' narratives of occupational identity. *American Journal of Occupational Therapy, 58*, 446–454.

Rebeiro, K. L., Day, D. G., Semeniuk, B., O'Brien, M. C., & Wilson, B. (2001). Northern Initiative for Social Action: An occupation-based mental

health program. *American Journal of Occupational Therapy, 55*, 493–500.

Reynolds, F. (2004). Textile art promoting well-being in long-term illness: Some general and specific influences. *Journal of Occupational Science, 11*, 58–67.

12. Successful performance in occupation can positively affect *psychological* functioning.

Case-Control and Cohort Designs

MacKinnon, J. R., & Miller, W. C. (2003). Rheumatoid arthritis and self-esteem: The impact of quality occupation. *Journal of Occupational Science, 10*, 90–98.

Case Studies

Legault, E., & Rebeiro, K. L. (2001). Occupation as means to mental health: A single case study. *American Journal of Occupational Therapy, 55*, 90–96.

Nonrandomized Research Designs

Smith, S. A., Press, B., Koenig, K. P., & Kinnealey, M. (2005). Effects of sensory integration intervention on self-stimulating and self-injurious behaviors. *American Journal of Occupational Therapy, 59*, 418–425.

Outcomes Research

Frank, G., Fishman, M., Crowley, C., Blair, B., Murphy, S. T., Montoya, J. A., et al. (2001). The New Stories/New Cultures after-school enrichment program: A direct cultural intervention. *American Journal of Occupational Therapy, 55*, 501–508.

Lysack, C. L., MacNeill, S. E., & Lichtenberg, P. A. (2001). The functional performance of elderly urban African-American women who return home to live alone after medical rehabilitation. *American Journal of Occupational Therapy, 55*, 433–440.

Oka, M., Otsuka, K., Yokoyama, N., Mintz, J., Hoshino, K., Niwa, S.-I., et al. (2004). An evaluation of a hybrid occupational therapy supported employment program in Japan for persons with schizophrenia. *American Journal of Occupational Therapy, 58*, 466–475.

Qualitative Research Designs

Camp, M. M. (2001). The use of service dogs as an adaptive strategy: A qualitative study. *American Journal of Occupational Therapy, 55,* 509–517.

Chan, S. C. C. (2004). Chronic obstructive pulmonary disease and engagement in occupation. *American Journal of Occupational Therapy, 58,* 408–415.

Howie, L., Coulter, M., & Feldman, S. (2004). Crafting the self: Older persons' narratives of occupational identity. *American Journal of Occupational Therapy, 58,* 446–454.

Mathiowetz, V., Finlayson, M. L., Matuska, K. M., Chen, H. Y., & Luo, P. (2005). Randomized control trial of an energy conservation course for persons with multiple sclerosis. *Multiple Sclerosis, 11,* 592–601.

Rebeiro, K. L., Day, D. G., Semeniuk, B., O'Brien, M. C., & Wilson, B. (2001). Northern Initiative for Social Action: An occupation-based mental health program. *American Journal of Occupational Therapy, 55,* 493–500.

Siporin, S., & Lysack, C. (2004). Quality of life and supported employment: A case study of three women with developmental disabilities. *American Journal of Occupational Therapy, 58,* 455–465.

Randomized Designs

Dooley, N. R., & Hinojosa, J. (2004). Improving quality of life for persons with Alzheimer's disease and their family caregivers: Brief occupational therapy intervention. *American Journal of Occupational Therapy, 58,* 561–569.

Norweg, A. M., Whiteson, J., Malgady, R., Mola, A., & Rey, M. (2005). The effectiveness of different combinations of pulmonary rehabilitation program components: A randomized control trial. *Chest, 128,* 663–672.

Shaffer, R. J., Jacokes, L. E., Cassily, J. F., Greenspan, S. I., Tuchman, R. F., & Temmer, P. J., Jr. (2001). Effect of interactive Metronome® training on children with ADHD. *American Journal of Occupational Therapy, 55,* 155–162.

Single-Case Designs

Holm, M. B., Santangelo, M. A., Fromuth, D. J., Brown, S. O., & Walter, H. (2000). Effectiveness of everyday occupations for changing client behaviors in a community living arrangement. *American Journal of Occupational Therapy, 54,* 361–371.

Melchert-McKearnan, K., Deitz, J., Engel, J. M., & White, O. (2000). Children with burn injuries: Purposeful activity versus rote exercise. *American Journal of Occupational Therapy, 54,* 381–390.

Systematic Evidence Reviews

Woods, B., Spector, A., Jones, C., Orrell, M., & Davies, S. (2005). Reminiscence therapy for dementia. *Cochrane Database of Systematic Reviews,* Issue 2, CD001120. DOI:10.1002/14651858.CD001120.pub2.

13. Occupations have unique *meaning and purpose* for each person, which influence the quality of performance (AOTA, 2002).

14. Engagement in occupations gives a sense of *satisfaction* and *fulfillment* (AOTA, 2002).

Case Studies

Legault, E., & Rebeiro, K. L. (2001). Occupation as means to mental health: A single case study. *American Journal of Occupational Therapy, 55,* 90–96.

Nonrandomized Designs

Jackson, J. P., & Schkade, J. K. (2001). Occupational adaptation model versus biomechanical–rehabilitation model in the treatment of patients with hip fractures. *American Journal of Occupational Therapy, 55,* 531–537.

Trombly, C. A., Radomski, M. V., Trexel, C., & Burnett-Smith, S. E. (2002). Occupational therapy and achievement of self-identified goals by adults with acquired brain injury: Phase II. *American Journal of Occupational Therapy, 56,* 489–498.

Outcomes Research

Frank, G., Fishman, M., Crowley, C., Blair, B., Murphy, S. T., Montoya, J. A., et al. (2001). The New Stories/New Cultures after-school enrichment program: A direct cultural intervention. *American Journal of Occupational Therapy, 55,* 501–508.

Qualitative Research Designs

Bontje, P., Kinébanian, A., Josephsson, S., & Tamura, Y. (2004). Occupational adaptation: The experiences of older persons with physical disabilities. *American Journal of Occupational Therapy, 58,* 140–149.

Rebeiro, K. L., Day, D. G., Semeniuk, B., O'Brien, M. C., & Wilson, B. (2001). Northern Initiative for Social Action: An occupation-based mental health program. *American Journal of Occupational Therapy, 55,* 493–500.

Randomized Designs

VanLeit, B., & Crowe, T. K. (2002). Outcomes of an occupational therapy program for mothers of children with disabilities: Impact on satisfaction with time use and occupational performance. *American Journal of Occupational Therapy, 56,* 402–410.

Systematic Reviews

Han, A., Judd, M. G., Robinson, V. A., Taixiang, W., Tugwell, P., & Wells, G. (2004). Tai chi for treating rheumatoid arthritis. *Cochrane Database of Systematic Reviews,* Issue 3, CD004849. DOI: 10.1002/14651858.CD004849.

15. Occupations influence how persons *spend time* and *make decisions* (AOTA, 2002).

Outcomes Research

Frank, G., Fishman, M., Crowley, C., Blair, B., Murphy, S. T., Montoya, J. A., et al. (2001). The New Stories/New Cultures after-school enrichment program: A direct cultural intervention. *American Journal of Occupational Therapy, 55,* 501–508.

Qualitative Research Designs

Chan, S. C. C. (2004). Chronic obstructive pulmonary disease and engagement in occupation. *American Journal of Occupational Therapy, 58,* 408–415.

Spencer, J., Hersch, G., Shelton, M., Ripple, J., Spencer, C., Dyer, C. B., et al. (2002). Functional outcomes and daily life activities of African-American elders after hospitalization. *American Journal of Occupational Therapy, 56,* 149–159.

Randomized Designs

VanLeit, B., & Crowe, T. K. (2002). Outcomes of an occupational therapy program for mothers of children with disabilities: Impact on satisfaction with time use and occupational performance. *American Journal of Occupational Therapy, 56,* 402–410.

Single-Case Designs

Holm, M. B., Santangelo, M. A., Fromuth, D. J., Brown, S. O., & Walter, H. (2000). Effectiveness of everyday occupations for changing client behaviors in a community living arrangement. *American Journal of Occupational Therapy, 54,* 361–371.

Appendix D

Guidelines for Supervision, Roles, and Responsibilities During the Delivery of Occupational Therapy Services

This document contains four sections that direct the delivery of occupational therapy services. These sections are The Guidelines for the Supervision of Occupational Therapy Personnel,[1] Supervision of Occupational Therapists and Occupational Therapy Assistants, Roles and Responsibilities of Occupational Therapists and Occupational Therapy Assistants During the Delivery of Occupational Therapy Services, and Supervision of Occupational Therapy Aides.

The Guidelines for the Supervision of Occupational Therapy Personnel

These guidelines provide a definition of supervision and outline parameters to be used by occupational therapy personnel regarding effective supervision as it relates to the delivery of occupational therapy services. These supervision guidelines are to assist occupational therapy personnel in the appropriate and effective provision of occupational therapy services. The guidelines themselves cannot be interpreted to constitute a standard of supervision in any particular locality. All personnel are expected to meet applicable state and federal regulations, adhere to relevant workplace policies and the *Occupational Therapy Code of Ethics* (AOTA, 2000), and participate in ongoing professional development activities to maintain continuing competency.

In these guidelines, supervision is viewed as a cooperative process in which two or more people participate in a joint effort to establish, maintain, and/or elevate a level of competence and perform-ance. Supervision is based on mutual understanding between the supervisor and the supervisee about each other's competence, experience, education, and credentials. It fosters growth and development, promotes effective utilization of resources, encourages creativity and innovation, and provides education and support to achieve a goal (AOTA, 1999a). Within the scope of occupational therapy practice, supervision is a process aimed at ensuring the safe and effective delivery of occupational therapy services and fostering professional competence and development.

Supervision of Occupational Therapists and Occupational Therapy Assistants

Occupational Therapists

Based on their education and training, occupational therapists, after initial certification, are autonomous practitioners who are able to deliver occupational therapy services independently. The occupational therapist is responsible for all aspects of occupational therapy service delivery and is accountable for the safety and effectiveness of the occupational therapy service delivery process. Occupational therapists are encouraged to seek supervision and mentoring to develop best practice approaches and promote professional growth.

Occupational Therapy Assistants

Based on their education and training, occupational therapy assistants must receive supervision from an occupational therapist to deliver occupational therapy services. The occupational therapy assistant delivers occupational therapy services under the supervision of and in partnership with the occupational therapist. The occupational therapist and the occupational therapy assistant are

---

[1]Occupational therapy personnel include occupational therapists, occupational therapy assistants, and occupational therapy aides (AOTA, 1999a).

responsible for collaboratively developing a plan for supervision.

General Principles

1. Supervision involves guidance and oversight related to the delivery of occupational therapy services and the facilitation of professional growth and competence. It is the responsibility of the occupational therapist and the occupational therapy assistant to seek the appropriate quality and frequency of supervision to ensure safe and effective occupational therapy service delivery.

2. To ensure safe and effective occupational therapy services, it is the responsibility of the occupational therapist and occupational therapy assistant to recognize when supervision is needed, and to seek supervision that supports current and advancing levels of competence.

3. The specific frequency, methods, and content of supervision may vary by practice setting and are dependent upon the
   a. Complexity of client needs,
   b. Number and diversity of clients,
   c. Skills of the occupational therapist and the occupational therapy assistant,
   d. Type of practice setting,
   e. Requirements of the practice setting, and
   f. Other regulatory requirements.

4. Supervision that is more frequent than the minimum level required by the practice setting or regulatory agencies may be necessary when
   a. The needs of the client and the occupational therapy process are complex and changing,
   b. The practice setting provides occupational therapy services to a large number of clients with diverse needs, or
   c. The occupational therapist and occupational therapy assistant determine that additional supervision is necessary to ensure safe and effective delivery of occupational therapy services.

5. A variety of types and methods of supervision should be used. Methods may include direct face-to-face contact and indirect contact. Examples of methods or types of supervision that involve direct face-to-face contact include observation, modeling, co-treatment, discussions, teaching, and instruction. Examples of methods or types of supervision that involve indirect contact include phone conversations, written correspondence, and electronic exchanges.

6. Occupational therapists and occupational therapy assistants must abide by agency and state requirements regarding the documentation of a supervision plan and supervision contacts. Documentation may include the
   a. Frequency of supervisory contact,
   b. Method(s) or type(s) of supervision,
   c. Content areas addressed,
   d. Evidence to support areas and levels of competency, and
   e. Names and credentials of the persons participating in the supervisory process.

7. Supervision related to professional growth, such as leadership and advocacy development, may differ from that needed to provide occupational therapy services. The person providing this supervision, as well as the frequency, method, and content of supervision, should be responsive to the supervisee's advancing levels of professional growth.

Supervision Outside the Delivery of Occupational Therapy Services

The education and expertise of occupational therapists and occupational therapy assistants prepare them for employment in arenas other than those related to the delivery of occupational therapy. In these other arenas, supervision may be provided by non-occupational therapy professionals.

1. The guidelines of the setting, regulatory agencies, and funding agencies direct the supervision requirements.

2. The occupational therapist and occupational therapy assistant should obtain and use credentials or job titles commensurate with their roles in these other employment arenas.

3. The following are used to determine whether the services provided are related to the delivery of occupational therapy:
   a. State practice acts

b. Regulatory agency standards and rules

c. The domain of occupational therapy practice

d. The written and verbal agreement among the occupational therapist, the occupational therapy assistant, the client, and the agency or payer about the services provided.

Roles and Responsibilities of Occupational Therapists and Occupational Therapy Assistants During the Delivery of Occupational Therapy Services

General Statement

The focus of occupational therapy is to facilitate the engagement of the client in occupations that support participation in daily life situations in context or contexts. Occupational therapy addresses the needs and goals of the client related to areas of occupation, performance skills, performance patterns, occupational context, activity demands, and client factors.

1. The occupational therapist is responsible for all aspects of occupational therapy service delivery and is accountable for the safety and effectiveness of the occupational therapy service delivery process. The occupational therapy service delivery process involves evaluation, intervention planning, intervention implementation, intervention review, and outcome evaluation.

2. The occupational therapist must be directly involved in the delivery of services during the initial evaluation and regularly throughout the course of intervention and outcome evaluation.

3. The occupational therapy assistant delivers occupational therapy services under the supervision of and in partnership with the occupational therapist.

4. It is the responsibility of the occupational therapist to determine when to delegate responsibilities to other occupational therapy personnel. It is the responsibility of the occupational therapy personnel who perform the delegated responsibilities to demonstrate service competency.

5. The occupational therapist and the occupational therapy assistant demonstrate and document service competency for clinical reasoning and judgment during the service delivery process as well as for the performance of specific techniques, assessments, and intervention methods used.

6. When delegating aspects of occupational therapy services, the occupational therapist considers the following factors:

a. The complexity of the client's condition and needs

b. The knowledge, skill, and competence of the occupational therapy practitioner

c. The nature and complexity of the intervention

d. The needs and requirements of the practice setting.

Roles and Responsibilities

Regardless of the setting in which occupational therapy services are delivered, the occupational therapist and the occupational therapy assistant assume the following generic responsibilities during evaluation, intervention, and outcomes evaluation.

Evaluation

1. The occupational therapist directs the evaluation process.

2. The occupational therapist is responsible for directing all aspects of the initial contact during the occupational therapy evaluation, including

a. Determining the need for service,

b. Defining the problems within the domain of occupational therapy that need to be addressed,

c. Determining the client's goals and priorities,

d. Establishing intervention priorities,

e. Determining specific further assessment needs, and

f. Determining specific assessment tasks that can be delegated to the occupational therapy assistant.

3. The occupational therapist initiates and directs the evaluation, interprets the data, and develops the intervention plan.

4. The occupational therapy assistant contributes to the evaluation process by implementing delegated assessments and by providing verbal and written reports of observations and client capacities to the occupational therapist.

5. The occupational therapist interprets the information provided by the occupational therapy assistant and integrates that information into the evaluation and decision-making process.

Intervention Planning

1. The occupational therapist has overall responsibility for the development of the occupational therapy intervention plan.

2. The occupational therapist and the occupational therapy assistant collaborate with the client to develop the plan.

3. The occupational therapy assistant is responsible for being knowledgeable about evaluation results and for providing input into the intervention plan, based on client needs and priorities.

Intervention Implementation

1. The occupational therapist has overall responsibility for implementing the intervention.

2. When delegating aspects of the occupational therapy intervention to the occupational therapy assistant, the occupational therapist is responsible for providing appropriate supervision.

3. The occupational therapy assistant is responsible for being knowledgeable about the client's occupational therapy goals.

4. The occupational therapy assistant selects, implements, and makes modifications to therapeutic activities and interventions that are consistent with demonstrated competency levels, client goals, and the requirements of the practice setting.

Intervention Review

1. The occupational therapist is responsible for determining the need for continuing, modifying, or discontinuing occupational therapy services.

2. The occupational therapy assistant contributes to this process by exchanging information with and providing documentation to the occupational therapist about the client's responses to and communications during intervention.

Outcome Evaluation

1. The occupational therapist is responsible for selecting, measuring, and interpreting outcomes that are related to the client's ability to engage in occupations.

2. The occupational therapy assistant is responsible for being knowledgeable about the client's targeted occupational therapy outcomes and for providing information and documentation related to outcome achievement.

3. The occupational therapy assistant may implement outcome measurements and provide needed client discharge resources.

Supervision of Occupational Therapy Aides[2]

An aide, as used in occupational therapy practice, is an individual who provides supportive services to the occupational therapist and the occupational therapy assistant. Aides are not primary service providers of occupational therapy in any practice setting. Therefore, aides do not provide skilled occupational therapy services. An aide is trained by an occupational therapist or an occupational therapy assistant to perform specifically delegated tasks. The occupational therapist is responsible for the overall use and actions of the aide. An aide first must demonstrate competency to be able to perform the assigned, delegated client and non-client tasks.

1. The occupational therapist must oversee the development, documentation, and implementation of a plan to supervise and routinely assess the ability of the occupational therapy aide to carry out non-client- and client-related tasks.

---

[2]Depending on the setting in which service is provided, aides may be referred to by various names. Examples include, but are not limited to, *rehabilitation aides, restorative aides, extenders, paraprofessionals,* and *rehab techs* (AOTA, 1999b).

The occupational therapy assistant may contribute to the development and documentation of this plan.

2. The occupational therapy assistant can supervise the aide.

3. Non-client-related tasks include clerical and maintenance activities and preparation of the work area or equipment.

4. Client-related tasks are routine tasks during which the aide may interact with the client but does not act as a primary service provider of occupational therapy services. The following factors must be present when an occupational therapist or occupational therapy assistant delegates a selected client-related task to the aide:

   a. The outcome anticipated for the delegated task is predictable.

   b. The situation of the client and the environment is stable and will not require that judgment, interpretations, or adaptations be made by the aide.

   c. The client has demonstrated some previous performance ability in executing the task.

   d. The task routine and process have been clearly established.

5. When performing delegated client-related tasks, the supervisor must ensure that the aide

   a. Is trained and able to demonstrate competency in carrying out the selected task and using equipment, if appropriate;

   b. Has been instructed on how to specifically carry out the delegated task with the specific client; and

   c. Knows the precautions, signs, and symptoms for the particular client that would indicate the need to seek assistance from the occupational therapist or occupational therapy assistant.

6. The supervision of the aide needs to be documented. Documentation includes information about frequency and methods of supervision used, the content of supervision, and the names and credentials of all persons participating in the supervisory process.

Summary

These guidelines about supervision, roles, and responsibilities are to assist in the appropriate utilization of occupational therapy personnel and in the appropriate and effective provision of occupational therapy services. All personnel are expected to meet applicable state and federal regulations, adhere to relevant workplace policies and the *Occupational Therapy Code of Ethics* (AOTA, 2000), and participate in ongoing professional development activities to maintain continuing competency.

References

American Occupational Therapy Association. (1999a). Guide for supervision of occupational therapy personnel in the delivery of occupational therapy services. *American Journal of Occupational Therapy, 53,* 592–594 [correction, 54(2): 235].

American Occupational Therapy Association. (1999b). Guidelines for the use of aides in occupational therapy practice. *American Journal of Occupational Therapy, 53,* 595–597 [correction, 54(2): 235].

American Occupational Therapy Association. (2000). Occupational therapy code of ethics. *American Journal of Occupational Therapy, 54,* 614–616.

Additional Reading

American Occupational Therapy Association. (1998). Standards of practice for occupational therapy. *American Journal of Occupational Therapy, 52,* 866–869.

American Occupational Therapy Association. (2002a). Parameters for appropriate supervision of the occupational therapy assistant. *OT Practice, 7*(15), 9.

American Occupational Therapy Association. (2002b). Roles and responsibilities of the occupational therapist and the occupational therapy assistant during the delivery of occupational therapy services. *OT Practice, 7*(15), 9–10.

Authors

The Commission on Practice:

Sara Jane Brayman, PhD, OTR/L, FAOTA,
 Chairperson

Gloria Frolek Clark, MS, OTR/L, FAOTA

Janet V. DeLany, DEd, OTR/L

Eileen R. Garza, PhD, OTR, ATP

Mary V. Radomski, MA, OTR/L, FAOTA

Ruth Ramsey, MS, OTR/L

Carol Siebert, MS, OTR/L

Kristi Voelkerding, BS, COTA/L

Pataricia D. LaVesser, PhD, OTR/L, *SIS Liaison*

Lenna Aird, ASD Liaison

Deborah Lieberman, MHSA, OTR/L, FAOTA, *AOTA
 Headquarters Liaison*

for

The Commission on Practice

Sara Jane Brayman, PhD, OTR/L, FAOTA,
 Chairperson

Adopted by the Representative Assembly 2004C24

This document replaces the following AOTA documents:

- 1999 *Guidelines for Use of Aides in Occupational Therapy Practice* (previously published and copyrighted in 1999 by the *American Journal of Occupational Therapy, 53,* 595–597 [correction, 54(2): 235]).

- 1999 *Guide for Supervision of Occupational Therapy Personnel in the Delivery of Occupational Therapy Services* (previously published and copyrighted in 1999 by the *American Journal of Occupational Therapy, 53,* 592–594 [correction, 54(2):235]).

- *2002 Parameters for Appropriate Supervision of the Occupational Therapy Assistant* (previously published and copyrighted by *OT Practice, 7*(15), 9).

- *2002 Roles and Responsibilities of the Occupational Therapist and the Occupational Therapy Assistant During the Delivery of Occupational Therapy Services* (previously published and copyrighted by *OT Practice, 7*(15), 9–10).

Appendix E | Standards of Practice for Occupational Therapy

Preface

This document defines minimum standards for the practice of occupational therapy. The *Standards of Practice for Occupational Therapy* are requirements for occupational therapists and occupational therapy assistants for the delivery of occupational therapy services. *The Reference Manual of Official Documents* contains documents that clarify and support occupational therapy practice (American Occupational Therapy Association [AOTA], 2004). These documents are reviewed and updated on an ongoing basis for their applicability.

Education, Examination, and Licensure Requirements

All occupational therapists and occupational therapy assistants must practice under federal and state law.

To practice as an occupational therapist, the individual trained in the United States

- Has graduated from an occupational therapy program accredited by the Accreditation Council for Occupational Therapy Education (ACOTE) or predecessor organizations;
- Has successfully completed a period of supervised fieldwork experience required by the recognized educational institution where the applicant met the academic requirements of an educational program for occupational therapists that is accredited by ACOTE or predecessor organizations;
- Has passed a nationally recognized entry-level examination for occupational therapists; and
- Fulfills state requirements for licensure, certification, or registration.

To practice as an occupational therapy assistant, the individual trained in the United States

- Has graduated from an associate- or certificate-level occupational therapy assistant program accredited by ACOTE or predecessor organizations;
- Has successfully completed a period of supervised fieldwork experience required by the recognized educational institution where the applicant met the academic requirements of an educational program for occupational therapy assistants that is accredited by ACOTE or predecessor organizations;
- Has passed a nationally recognized entry-level examination for occupational therapy assistants; and
- Fulfills state requirements for licensure, certification, or registration.

Definitions

Assessment
Specific tools or instruments that are used during the evaluation process.

Client
A person, group, program, organization, or community for whom the occupational therapy practitioner is providing services.

Evaluation
The process of obtaining and interpreting data necessary for intervention. This includes planning for and documenting the evaluation process and results.

Screening
Obtaining and reviewing data relevant to a potential client to determine the need for further evaluation and intervention.

Standard I: Professional Standing and Responsibility

1. An occupational therapy practitioner (occupational therapist or occupational therapy assistant) delivers occupational therapy services that reflect the philosophical base of occupational therapy and are consistent with the established principles and concepts of theory and practice.
2. An occupational therapy practitioner is knowledgeable about and delivers occupational therapy services in accordance with AOTA standards, policies, and guidelines and state and federal requirements relevant to practice and service delivery.
3. An occupational therapy practitioner maintains current licensure, registration, or certification as required by law or regulation.
4. An occupational therapy practitioner abides by the AOTA *Occupational Therapy Code of Ethics* (AOTA, 2000).
5. An occupational therapy practitioner abides by the AOTA *Standards for Continuing Competence* (AOTA, 1999) by establishing, maintaining, and updating professional performance, knowledge, and skills.
6. An occupational therapist is responsible for all aspects of occupational therapy service delivery and is accountable for the safety and effectiveness of the occupational therapy service delivery process.
7. An occupational therapy assistant is responsible for providing safe and effective occupational therapy services under the supervision of and in partnership with the occupational therapist and in accordance with laws or regulations and AOTA documents.
8. An occupational therapy practitioner maintains current knowledge of legislative, political, social, cultural, and reimbursement issues that affect clients and the practice of occupational therapy.
9. An occupational therapy practitioner is knowledgeable about evidence-based research and applies it ethically and appropriately to the occupational therapy process.

Standard II: Screening, Evaluation, and Re-evaluation

1. An occupational therapist accepts and responds to referrals in compliance with state laws or other regulatory requirements.
2. An occupational therapist, in collaboration with the client, evaluates the client's ability to participate in daily life activities by considering the client's capacities, the activities, and the environments in which these activities occur.
3. An occupational therapist initiates and directs the screening, evaluation, and re-evaluation process and analyzes and interprets the data in accordance with law, regulatory requirements, and AOTA documents.
4. An occupational therapy assistant contributes to the screening, evaluation, and re-evaluation process by implementing delegated assessments and by providing verbal and written reports of observations and client capacities to the occupational therapist in accordance with law, regulatory requirements, and AOTA documents.
5. An occupational therapy practitioner follows defined protocols when standardized assessments are used.
6. An occupational therapist completes and documents occupational therapy evaluation results. An occupational therapy assistant contributes to the documentation of evaluation results. An occupational therapy practitioner abides by the time frames, formats, and standards established by practice settings, government agencies, external accreditation programs, payers, and AOTA documents.
7. An occupational therapy practitioner communicates screening, evaluation, and re-evaluation results within the boundaries of client confidentiality to the appropriate person, group, or organization.
8. An occupational therapist recommends additional consultations or refers clients to appropriate resources when the needs of the client can best be served by the expertise of other professionals or services.

9. An occupational therapy practitioner educates current and potential referral sources about the scope of occupational therapy services and the process of initiating occupational therapy services.

Standard III: Intervention

1. An occupational therapist has overall responsibility for the development, documentation, and implementation of the occupational therapy intervention based on the evaluation, client goals, current best evidence, and clinical reasoning.

2. An occupational therapist ensures that the intervention plan is documented within the time frames, formats, and standards established by the practice settings, agencies, external accreditation programs, and payers.

3. An occupational therapy assistant selects, implements, and makes modifications to therapeutic activities and interventions that are consistent with the occupational therapy assistant's demonstrated competency and delegated responsibilities, the intervention plan, and requirements of the practice setting.

4. An occupational therapy practitioner reviews the intervention plan with the client and appropriate others regarding the rationale, safety issues, and relative benefits and risks of the planned interventions.

5. An occupational therapist modifies the intervention plan throughout the intervention process and documents changes in the client's needs, goals, and performance.

6. An occupational therapy assistant contributes to the modification of the intervention plan by exchanging information with and providing documentation to the occupational therapist about the client's responses to and communications throughout the intervention.

7. An occupational therapy practitioner documents the occupational therapy services provided within the time frames, formats, and standards established by the practice settings, agencies,

external accreditation programs, payers, and AOTA documents.

Standard IV: Outcomes

1. An occupational therapist is responsible for selecting, measuring, documenting, and interpreting expected or achieved outcomes that are related to the client's ability to engage in occupations.

2. An occupational therapist is responsible for documenting changes in the client's performance and capacities and for discontinuing services when the client has achieved identified goals, reached maximum benefit, or does not desire to continue services.

3. An occupational therapist prepares and implements a discontinuation plan or transition plan based on the client's needs, goals, performance, and appropriate follow-up resources.

4. An occupational therapy assistant contributes to the discontinuation or transition plan by providing information and documentation to the supervising occupational therapist related to the client's needs, goals, performance, and appropriate follow-up resources.

5. An occupational therapy practitioner facilitates the transition process in collaboration with the client; family members; significant others; team; and community resources and individuals, when appropriate.

6. An occupational therapist is responsible for evaluating the safety and effectiveness of the occupational therapy processes and interventions within the practice setting.

7. An occupational therapy assistant contributes to evaluating the safety and effectiveness of the occupational therapy processes and interventions within the practice setting.

References

American Occupational Therapy Association. (1999). Standards for continuing competence. *American Journal of Occupational Therapy, 53,* 599–600.

American Occupational Therapy Association. (2000). Occupational therapy code of ethics (2000). *American Journal of Occupational Therapy, 54,* 614–616.

American Occupational Therapy Association. (2004). *The reference manual of the official documents of the American Occupational Therapy Association* (10th ed.). Bethesda, MD: Author.

Authors

The Commission on Practice

Sara Jane Brayman, PhD, OTR/L, FAOTA,
  Chairperson

Susanne Smith Roley, MS, OTR/L, FAOTA,
  Chairperson-Elect

Gloria Frolek Clark, MS, OTR/L, FAOTA

Janet V. DeLany, DEd, MSA, OTR/L, FAOTA

Eileen R. Garza, PhD, OTR, ATP

Mary V. Radomski, MA, OTR/L, FAOTA

Ruth Ramsey, MS, OTR/L

Carol Siebert, MS, OTR/L

Kristi Voelkerding, BS, COTA/L

Lenna Aird, COTA/L, *ASD Liaison*

Patricia D. LaVesser, PhD, OTR/L, *SIS Liaison*

Deborah Lieberman, MHSA, OTR/L, FAOTA, AOTA
  Headquarters Liaison

for

The Commission on Practice

Sara Jane Brayman, PhD, OTR/L, FAOTA,
  Chairperson

Adopted by the Representative Assembly 2005C218

Note: This document replaces the 1998 *Standards of Practice for Occupational Therapy.* These standards are intended as recommended guidelines to assist occupational therapy practitioners in the provision of occupational therapy services. These standards serve as a minimum standard for occupational therapy practice and are applicable to all individual populations and the programs in which these individuals are served.

Appendix F | Occupational Therapy Code of Ethics (2005)

Preamble

The American Occupational Therapy Association (AOTA) *Occupational Therapy Code of Ethics* (2005) is a public statement of principles used to promote and maintain high standards of conduct within the profession and is supported by the *Core Values and Attitudes of Occupational Therapy Practice* (AOTA, 1993). Members of AOTA are committed to promoting inclusion, diversity, independence, and safety for all recipients in various stages of life, health, and illness and to empower all beneficiaries of occupational therapy. This commitment extends beyond service recipients to include professional colleagues, students, educators, businesses, and the community.

Fundamental to the mission of the occupational therapy profession is the therapeutic use of everyday life activities (occupations) with individuals or groups for the purpose of participation in roles and situations in home, school, workplace, community, and other settings. "Occupational therapy addresses the physical, cognitive, psychosocial, sensory, and other aspects of performance in a variety of contexts to support engagement in everyday life activities that affect health, well-being and quality of life" (*Definition of Occupational Therapy Practice for the AOTA Model Practice Act*, 2004). Occupational therapy personnel have an ethical responsibility first and foremost to recipients of service as well as to society.

The historical foundation of this Code is based on ethical reasoning surrounding practice and professional issues, as well as empathic reflection regarding these interactions with others. This reflec-tion resulted in the establishment of principles that guide ethical action. Ethical action goes beyond rote following of rules or application of principles; rather, it is a manifestation of moral character and mindful reflection. It is a commitment to benefi-cence for the sake of others, to virtuous practice of artistry and science, to genuinely good behaviors, and to noble acts of courage. It is an empathic way of being among others, which is made every day by all occupational therapy personnel.

The AOTA *Occupational Therapy Code of Ethics* (2005) is an aspirational guide to professional conduct when ethical issues surface. Ethical decision making is a process that includes awareness regarding how the outcome will impact occupational therapy clients in all spheres. Applications of Code principles are considered situation-specific, and where a conflict exists, occupational therapy personnel will pursue responsible efforts for resolution.

The specific purpose of the AOTA *Occupational Therapy Code of Ethics* (2005) is to:

1. Identify and describe the principles supported by the occupational therapy profession
2. Educate the general public and members regarding established principles to which occupational therapy personnel are accountable
3. Socialize occupational therapy personnel new to the practice to expected standards of conduct
4. Assist occupational therapy personnel in recognition and resolution of ethical dilemmas.

The AOTA *Occupational Therapy Code of Ethics* (2005) defines the set principles that apply to occupational therapy personnel at all levels:

Principle 1. Occupational therapy personnel shall demonstrate a concern for the safety and well-being of the recipients of their services. (Beneficence)

Occupational therapy personnel shall

A. Provide services in a fair and equitable manner. They shall recognize and appreciate the cultural components of economics, geography, race, ethnicity, religious and political factors, marital status, age, sexual orientation, gender identity, and disability of all recipients of their services.

B. Strive to ensure that fees are fair and reasonable and commensurate with services performed. When occupational therapy practitioners set fees, they shall set fees considering institutional, local, state, and federal requirements, and with due regard for the service recipient's ability to pay.

C. Make every effort to advocate for recipients to obtain needed services through available means.

D. Recognize the responsibility to promote public health and the safety and well-being of individuals, groups, and/or communities.

Principle 2. Occupational therapy personnel shall take measures to ensure a recipient's safety and avoid imposing or inflicting harm. (Nonmaleficence)

Occupational therapy personnel shall

A. Maintain therapeutic relationships that shall not exploit the recipient of services sexually, physically, emotionally, psychologically, financially, socially, or in any other manner.

B. Avoid relationships or activities that conflict or interfere with therapeutic professional judgment and objectivity.

C. Refrain from any undue influences that may compromise provision of service.

D. Exercise professional judgment and critically analyze directives that could result in potential harm before implementation.

E. Identify and address personal problems that may adversely impact professional judgment and duties.

F. Bring concerns regarding impairment of professional skills of a colleague to the attention of the appropriate authority when or if attempts to address concerns are unsuccessful.

Principle 3. Occupational therapy personnel shall respect recipients to assure their rights. (Autonomy, Confidentiality)

Occupational therapy personnel shall

A. Collaborate with recipients, and if theydesire, families, significant others, and/or caregivers in setting goals and priorities throughout the intervention process, including full disclosure of the nature, risk, and potential outcomes of any interventions.

B. Obtain informed consent from participants involved in research activities and ensure that they understand potential risks and outcomes.

C. Respect the individual's right to refuse professional services or involvement in research or educational activities.

D. Protect all privileged confidential forms of written, verbal, and electronic communication gained from educational, practice, research, and investigational activities unless otherwise mandated by local, state, or federal regulations.

Principle 4. Occupational therapy personnel shall achieve and continually maintain high standards of competence. (Duty)

Occupational therapy personnel shall

A. Hold the appropriate national, state, or any other requisite credentials for the services they provide.

B. Conform to AOTA standards of practice and official documents.

C. Take responsibility for maintaining and documenting competence in practice, education, and research by participating in professional development and educational activities.

D. Be competent in all topic areas in which they provide instruction to consumers, peers, and/or students.

E. Critically examine available evidence so they may perform their duties on the basis of current information.

F. Protect service recipients by ensuring that duties assumed by or assigned to other occupational therapy personnel match credentials, qualifications, experience, and scope of practice.

G. Provide appropriate supervision to individuals for whom they have supervisory responsibility in accordance with Association official documents; local, state, and federal or national laws and regulations; and institutional policies and procedures.

H. Refer to or consult with other service providers whenever such a referral or consultation would be helpful to the care of the recipient of service. The referral or consultation process shall be done in collaboration with the recipient of service.

Principle 5. Occupational therapy personnel shall comply with laws and Association policies guiding the profession of occupational therapy. (Procedural Justice)

Occupational therapy personnel shall

A. Familiarize themselves with and seek to understand and abide by institutional rules; applicable Association policies; and local, state, and federal/national/international laws.

B. Be familiar with revisions in those laws and Association policies that apply to the profession of occupational therapy and shall inform employers, employees, and colleagues of those changes.

C. Encourage those they supervise in occupational therapy–related activities to adhere to the Code.

D. Take reasonable steps to ensure employers are aware of occupational therapy's ethical obligations, as set forth in this Code, and of the impli-

cations of those obligations for occupational therapy practice, education, and research.

E. Record and report in an accurate and timely manner all information related to professional activities.

Principle 6. Occupational therapy personnel shall provide accurate information when representing the profession. (Veracity)

Occupational therapy personnel shall

A. Represent their credentials, qualifications, education, experience, training, and competence accurately. This is of particular importance for those to whom occupational therapy personnel provide their services or with whom occupational therapy personnel have a professional relationship.

B. Disclose any professional, personal, financial, business, or volunteer affiliations that may pose a conflict of interest to those with whom they may establish a professional, contractual, or other working relationship.

C. Refrain from using or participating in the use of any form of communication that contains false, fraudulent, deceptive, or unfair statements or claims.

D. Identify and fully disclose to all appropriate persons errors that compromise recipients' safety.

E. Accept responsibility for their professional actions that reduce the public's trust in occupational therapy services and those that perform those services.

Principle 7. Occupational therapy personnel shall treat colleagues and other professionals with respect, fairness, discretion, and integrity. (Fidelity)

Occupational therapy personnel shall

A. Preserve, respect, and safeguard confidential information about colleagues and staff, unless otherwise mandated by national, state, or local laws.

B. Accurately represent the qualifications, views, contributions, and findings of colleagues.

C. Take adequate measures to discourage, prevent, expose, and correct any breaches of the Code and report any breaches of the Code to the appropriate authority.

D. Avoid conflicts of interest and conflicts of commitment in employment and volunteer roles.

E. Use conflict resolution and/or alternative dispute resolution resources to resolve organizational and interpersonal conflicts.

F. Familiarize themselves with established policies and procedures for handling concerns about this Code, including familiarity with national, state, local, district, and territorial procedures for handling ethics complaints. These include policies and procedures created by AOTA, licensing and regulatory bodies, employers, agencies, certification boards, and other organizations having jurisdiction over occupational therapy practice.

Glossary

Autonomy

The right of an individual to self-determination.The ability to independently act on one's decisions for one's own well-being (Beau-champ & Childress, 2001).

Beneficence

Doing good for others or bringing about good for them. The duty to confer benefits to others.

Confidentiality

Not disclosing data or information that should be kept private to prevent harm and to abide by policies, regulations, and laws.

Dilemma

A situation in which one moral conviction or right action conflicts with another. It exists because there is no one, clear-cut, right answer.

Duty

Actions required of professionals by society or actions that are self-imposed.

Ethics

A systematic study of morality (i.e., rules of conduct that are grounded in philosophical principles and theory).

Fidelity

Faithfully fulfilling vows and promises, agreements, and discharging fiduciary responsibilities (Beauchamp & Childress, 2001).

Justice

Three types of justice are

• **Compensatory justice**—Making reparation for wrongs that have been done.

• **Distributive justice**—The act of distributing goods and burdens among members of society.

• **Procedural justice**—Assuring that processes are organized in a fair manner and policies or laws are followed.

Morality

Personal beliefs regarding values, rules, and principles of what is right or wrong. Morality may be culture-based or culture-driven.

Nonmaleficence

Not harming or causing harm to be done to oneself or others; the duty to ensure that no harm is done.
Veracity
A duty to tell the truth; avoid deception.

References

American Occupational Therapy Association. (1993). Core values and attitudes of occupational therapy practice. *American Journal of Occupational Therapy, 47*, 1085–1086.

American Occupational Therapy Association. (1998). Guidelines to the occupational therapy code of ethics. *American Journal of Occupational Therapy, 52,* 881–884.

American Occupational Therapy Association. (2004). Association policies. *American Journal of Occupational Therapy, 58,* 694–695.

Beauchamp, T. L., & Childress, J. F. (2001). *Principles of biomedical ethics* (5th ed.). New York: Oxford University Press.

Definition of Occupational Therapy Practice forthe AOTA Model Practice Act. (2004). Retrieved April 9, 2005, from www.aota.org/members/area4/docs/defotpractice.pdf

Authors

Commission on Standards and Ethics (SEC):

S. Maggie Reitz, PhD, OTR/L, FAOTA, *Chairperson*

Melba Arnold, MS, OTR/L

Linda Gabriel Franck, PhD, OTR/L

Darryl J. Austin, MS, OT/L

Diane Hill, COTA/L, AP, ROH

Lorie J. McQuade, MEd, CRC

Daryl K. Knox, MD

Deborah Yarett Slater, MS, OT/L, FAOTA, *Staff Liaison*

With contributions to the Preamble by Suzanne Peloquin, PhD, OTR, FAOTA

Adopted by the RepresentativeAssembly 2005C202
Note. This document replaces the 2000 document, *Occupational Therapy Code of Ethics* (2000) (*American Journal of Occupational Therapy, 54,* 614–616).

Prepared 4/7/2000, revised draft 1/2005, second revision 4/2005 by SEC.

Note: Commission on Standards and Ethics (SEC) changed to Ethics Commission (EC) in September 2005 per AOTA Bylaws.

Note. This *AOTA Occupational Therapy Code of Ethics* is one of three documents that constitute the "Ethics Standards." The other two are the *Core Values and Attitudes of Occupational Therapy Practice* (1993) and the *Guidelines to the Occupational Therapy Code of Ethics.*

Appendix G | Procedural Terminology (Coding Language)

The following list of procedural terminology provides a structure for associating occupational therapy client factors and interventions to coding terminology commonly used by third-party payers.[1] Readers should refer to the Medicine section of the most recent *Current Procedural Terminology (CPT™)*[2] to determine the proper codes and nomenclature for billing occupational therapy intervention. The American Medical Association annually updates the *CPT* codes and the corresponding general instructions for how to use them.

Terminology Related to the Evaluation Process

Occupational therapy evaluation and occupational therapy reevaluation

Orthotics management (assessment)

Wheelchair management (assessment)

Physical performance test or measurement (e.g., musculoskeletal functional capacity) Assistive technology assessment

Evaluation of oral and pharyngeal swallowing function

Motion fluoroscopic evaluation of swallowing

Flexible fiberoptic endoscopic evaluation of swallowing

Manual muscle testing

Terminology Related to Intervention (e.g., Remediation/Restoration, Compensation)

Therapeutic activities to improve functional performance

Self-care/home management training (e.g., activities of daily living, use of assistive technology, safety procedures)

Community/work reintegration training (e.g., transportation/driving, work environment modification)

Orthotics and prosthetic fitting and training

Wheelchair management (fitting, training)

Development of cognitive skills to improve attention, memory, problem solving

Treatment of swallowing dysfunction and/or oral function for feeding

Therapeutic exercises for strength and endurance, range of motion, and flexibility

Reeducation of movement, balance, coordination, kinesthetic sense, posture, and proprioception

Aquatic therapy with therapeutic exercise

Sensory integrative activities

Work hardening/conditioning

Development of cognitive skills through compensatory training

Physical Agent Modalities and Adjunct Procedures to Facilitate Engagement in Occupation

Heat or cold (ice or hot packs, paraffin bath, whirlpool, contrast baths)

Electrical stimulation or iontophoresis

Vasopneumatic devices

Ultrasound or phonophoresis

---

[1]No inference should be made regarding payer recognition of or payment for the services listed. Limitations on coverage of one or more of these services by occupational therapists may be defined by state regulation or established by individual payer policy.

[2]*CPT* is a trademark of the American Medical Association.

Biofeedback training
Massage Manual therapy techniques (myofascial
    release/soft tissue mobilization, manual lym-
    phatic drainage)
Wound care management

References

Agency for Health Research and Quality. (2000). *Outcomes research* [Fact Sheet] (AHRQ Pub. No. 00-P011.) Rockville, MD: Author. Retrieved from www.ahrq.gov/clinic/outfact.htm.

American Occupational Therapy Association. (1979). The philosophical base of occupational therapy. *American Journal of Occupational Therapy, 33,* 785.

American Occupational Therapy Association. (1994). Statement of occupational therapy referral. *American Journal of Occupational Therapy, 48,* 1034.

American Occupational Therapy Association. (1995). Position Paper—Occupational performance: Occupational therapy's definition of function. *American Journal of Occupational Therapy, 49,* 1015–1018.

American Occupational Therapy Association. (1999a). The guide to occupational therapy practice. *American Journal of Occupational Therapy, 53,* 245–322.

American Occupational Therapy Association. (1999b). Standards for an accredited educational program for the occupational therapist. *American Journal of Occupational Therapy, 53,* 575–582.

American Occupational Therapy Association. (1999c). Standards for an accredited educational program for the occupational therapy assistant. *American Journal of Occupational Therapy, 53,* 583–589.

American Occupational Therapy Association. (2002). Occupational therapy practice framework: Domain and process. *American Journal of Occupational Therapy, 56,* 609–639.

American Occupational Therapy Association. (2003). Policy 5.3: Licensure. *Policy manual.* Bethesda, MD: Author.

American Occupational Therapy Association. (2004a). *Definition of occupational therapy practice for the AOTA Model Practice Act.* Bethesda, MD: Author. Available from the State Affairs Group, American Occupational Therapy Association, 4720 Montgomery Lane, PO Box 31220, Bethesda, MD 20824-1220.

American Occupational Therapy Association (2004b). Guidelines for supervision, roles, and responsibilities during the delivery of occupational therapy services. *American Journal of Occupational Therapy, 58,* 663–667.

American Occupational Therapy. (2004c). Scope of practice. *American Journal of Occupational Therapy, 58,* 673–677.

American Occupational Therapy Association. (2005a). Occupational therapy code of ethics. *American Journal of Occupational Therapy, 59,* 639–642.

American Occupational Therapy Association. (2005b). Standards for continuing competence. *American Journal of Occupational Therapy, 59,* 661–662.

American Occupational Therapy Association. (2005c). Standards of practice for occupational therapy. *American Journal of Occupational Therapy, 59,* 663–665.

Barker, D., Reid, D., & Cott, C. (2004). Acceptance and meaning of wheelchair use in senior stroke survivors. *American Journal of Occupational Therapy, 58,* 221–230.

Bass-Haugen, J., Henderson, M. L., Larson, B. A., & Matuska, K. (2005). Occupational issues of concern in populations. In C. H. Christiansen & C. M. Baum (Eds.), *Occupational therapy performance, participation, and well-being.* Thorofare, NJ: Slack.

Baum, C. M., Bass-Haugen, J., & Christiansen, C. H. (2005). Person–environment–occupation–

performance: A model for planning interventions for individuals and organizations. In C. H. Christiansen & C. M. Baum (Eds.), *Occupational therapy performance, participation, and well-being* (pp. 338–371). Thorofare, NJ: Slack.

Baum, C. M., & Christiansen, C. H. (2005a). Outcomes: The results of interventions in occupational therapy practice. In C. H. Christiansen & C. M. Baum (Eds.), *Occupational therapy performance, participation, and well-being* (pp. 523–534). Thorofare, NJ: Slack.

Baum, C. M., & Christiansen, C. H. (2005b). Person–environment–occupation performance: An occupation-based framework for practice. In C. H. Christiansen & C. M. Baum (Eds.), *Occupational therapy performance, participation, and well-being* (pp. 243–259). Thorofare, NJ: Slack.

Berkeland, R., & Flinn, N. (2005). Therapy as learning. In C. H. Christiansen & C. M. Baum (Eds.), *Occupational therapy performance, participation, and well-being* (pp. 420–449). Thorofare, NJ: Slack.

Bontje, P., Kinebanian, A., Josephsson, S., & Tamura, Y. (2004). Occupational adaptation: the experiences of older persons with physical disabilities. *American Journal of Occupational Therapy, 58,* 140–149.

Burke, J. P. (2003). Philosophical basis of human occupation. In P. Kramer, J. Hinojosa, & C. B. Royeen (Eds.), *Perspectives in human occupation* (pp. 32–44). Baltimore, MD: Lippincott, Williams, & Wilkins.

Chan, J., & Spencer, J. (2004). Adaptation to hand injury: An evolving experience. *American Journal of Occupational Therapy, 58,* 128–139.

Christiansen, C. H. (1999). Defining lives: Occupation as identity: An essay on competence, coherence, and the creation of meaning. *American Journal of Occupational Therapy, 53,* 547–558.

Christiansen, C. H. (2005). Time use and patterns of occupation. In C. H. Christiansen & C. M. Baum (Eds.), *Occupational therapy performance, participation, and well-being* (pp. 71–83). Thorofare, NJ: Slack.

Christiansen, C. H., & Baum, C. M. (2005). The complexity of human occupation. In C. H. Christiansen & C. M. Baum (Eds.), *Occupational*

therapy performance, participation, and well-being (pp. 3–17). Thorofare, NJ: Slack.

Christiansen, C. H., & Matuska, K. M. (2004). The importance of everyday activities. In Christiansen, C. H., & Matuska, K. M. (Eds.). *Ways of living: Adaptive strategies for special needs* (3rd ed, pp. 1–20). Bethesda, MD: AOTA Press.

Clark, F., Azen, S. P., Carlson, M., Labree, M. D., & Hay, J. (2001). Embedding health promoting changes into the daily lives of independent-living older adults: Long-term follow-up of occupational therapy intervention. *Journal of Gerontology: Psychological Sciences, 56,* 60–63.

Clark, F., Azen, S. P., Zemke, R., Jackson, J., Carlson, M., Mandel, D., et al. (1997). Occupational therapy for independent-living older adults: A randomized controlled trial. *Journal of the American Medical Association, 278,* 1321–1326.

Crepeau, E. B. (2003). Analyzing occupation and activity: A way of thinking about occupational performance. In E. B. Crepeau, E. S. Cohn, & B. A. B. Schell (Eds.), *Willard and Spackman's occupational therapy* (10th ed., pp. 198–202). Philadelphia: Lippincott Williams & Wilkins.

Dale, L. (2004). Partnering with management to implement ergonomics in the industrial setting. *Work: A Journal of Prevention, Assessment, and Rehabilitation, 22,* 117–124.

Deitz, J., Swinth, Y., & White, O. (2002). Powered mobility and preschoolers with complex developmental delays. *American Journal of Occupational Therapy, 56,* 86–96.

Dolecheck, J., & Schkade, J. (1999). The extent dyna-mic standing endurance is affected when CVA subjects perform personally meaningful activities rather than nonmeaningful tasks. *Occupational Therapy Journal of Research, 19*(1), 40–54.

Epstein, C. F., & Jaffe, E. G. (2003). Consultation: Collaborative interventions for change. In G. L. McCormack, E. G. Jaffe, & M. Goodman-Lavey (Eds.), *The occupational therapy manager* (4th ed., pp. 259–286). Bethesda, MD: AOTA Press.

Erikson, A., Karlsson, G., Söderström, M., & Tham, K. (2004). A training apartment with electronic aids to daily living: Lived experiences of persons with brain damage. *American Journal of Occupational Therapy, 58,* 261–271.

Fazio, L. S. (2001). *Developing occupation-centered programs for the community: A workbook for students and professionals.* Upper Saddle River, NJ: Prentice Hall.

Fricke, J., & Unsworth, C. (2001). Time use and importance of instrumental activities of daily living. *Australian Occupational Therapy Journal, 48,* 118–131.

Gahnstrom-Strandqvist, K., Liukko, A., & Tham, K. (2003). The meaning of the working cooperative for persons with long-term mental illness: A phenomenological study. *American Journal of Occupational Therapy, 57,* 262–272.

Gasser-Wieland, T., & Rice, M. (2002). Occupational embeddedness during a reaching and placing task with survivors of cerebral vascular accident. *OTJR: Occupation, Participation, and Health, 22*(4), 153–160.

Giles, G. M. (2003). Starting up a new program, business, or practice. In G. L. McCormack, E. G. Jaffe, & M. Goodman-Lavey (Eds.), *The occupational therapy manager* (4th ed., pp. 193–218). Bethesda, MD: AOTA Press.

Goldberg, B., Brintnell, E., & Goldberg, J. (2002). The relationship between engagement in meaningful activities and quality of life in persons disabled by mental illness. *Occupational Therapy in Mental Health, 18*(2), 17–44.

Haglund, L., & Henriksson, C. (2003). Concepts in occupational therapy in relation to the ICF. *Occupational Therapy International, 10*(4), 253–268.

Handley-More, D., Deitz, J., Billingsley, F. L., & Coggins, T. (2003). Facilitating written work using computer word processing and word prediction. *American Journal of Occupational Therapy, 57,* 139–151.

Hay, J., LaBree, L., Luo, R., Clark, F., Carlson, M., Mandel, D., et al. (2002). Cost-effectiveness of preventive occupational therapy for independent-living older adults. *Journal of the American Geriatric Society, 50,* 1381–1388.

Hinojosa, J., & Kramer, P. (Eds.). (1998). *Occupational therapy evaluation of clients: Obtaining and interpreting data.* Bethesda, MD: American Occupational Therapy Association.

Holm, M., Rogers, J. C., & Stone, R. G. (2003). Person–task–environment interventions: A decision-making guide. In E. B. Crepeau, E. S. Cohn, & B. A. B. Schell (Eds.), *Willard and Spackman's occupational therapy* (10th ed., pp. 460–490). Philadelphia: Lippincott Williams & Wilkins.

Holm, M., Santangelo, M., Fromuth, D., Brown, S., & Walter, H. (2000). Effectiveness of everyday occupations for changing client behaviors in a community living arrangement. *American Journal of Occupational Therapy, 54,* 361–371.

Jackson, J., & Schkade, J. (2001). Occupational adaptation model versus biomechanical rehabilitation model in the treatment of patients with hip fractures. *American Journal of Occupational Therapy, 55,* 531–537.

Kazdin, A. E. (2003). *Research design in clinical psychology* (4th ed.). Boston: Allyn & Bacon.

Kielhofner, G. (2002). *A model of human occupation: Theory and application* (3rd ed.). Baltimore, MD: Lippincott Williams & Wilkins.

Kielhofner, G. (2004). *Conceptual foundations of occupational therapy* (3rd ed.). Philadelphia: F. A. Davis.

Kielhofner, G., Hammel, J., Finlayson, M., Helfrich, C., & Taylor, R. R. (2004). Documenting outcomes of occupational therapy: The Center for Outcomes Research and Education. *American Journal of Occupational Therapy, 58,* 15–23.

Kramer, P., & Hinojosa, J. (2000). Activity synthesis. In J. Hinojosa & M. L. Blount (Eds.), *The texture of life: Purposeful activities in occupational therapy* (pp. 91–105). Bethesda, MD: AOTA Press.

Law, M. (2002a). *Evidence-based rehabilitation: A guide to practice.* Thorofare, NJ: Slack.

Law, M. (2002b). Participation in the occupations of everyday life. *American Journal of Occupational Therapy, 56,* 640–649.

Lindberg, L., & Iwarsson, S. (2002). Subjective quality of life, health, I-ADL ability and adaptation strategies in fibromyalgia. *Clinical Rehabilitation, 16,* 675–683.

Moyers, P. A. (1999). The guide to occupational therapy practice. *American Journal of Occupational Therapy, 53,* 247–322.

Moyers, P. A. (2005). Introduction to occupation-based practice. In C. H. Christiansen & C. M. Baum (Eds.), *Occupational therapy performance, participation, and well-being* (pp. 220–241). Thorofare, NJ: Slack.

Moyers, P. A., & Christiansen, C. H. (2004). Planning intervention. In C. H. Christiansen & K. M. Matuska (Eds.), *Ways of living: Adaptive strategies for special needs* (3rd ed., pp. 71–83). Bethesda, MD: AOTA Press.

Neistadt, M. E., & Crepeau, E. B. (1998). Introduction to occupational therapy. In M. E. Neistadt & E. B. Crepeau (Eds.), *Willard and Spackman's occupational therapy* (9th ed., pp. 5–12). Philadelphia: Lippincott.

Nelson, D. L., & Jepson-Thomas, J. (2003). Occupational form, occupational performance, and a conceptual framework for therapeutic occupation. In P. Kramer, J. Hinojosa, & C. B. Royeen (Eds.) *Perspectives in human occupation participation in life* (pp. 87–155). Philadelphia: Lippincott Williams & Wilkins.

Ottenbacher, K. J., Tickle-Degnen, L., & Hasselkus, B. R. (2002). From the desk of the editor—Therapists awake! The challenge of evidence-based occupational therapy. *American Journal of Occupational Therapy, 56,* 247–249.

Peloquin, S. M. (2003). Spirituality: Meanings related to occupational therapy. In E. B. Crepeau, E. S. Cohn, & B. A. B. Schell (Eds.), *Willard and Spackman's occupational therapy* (10th ed., pp. 121–126). Philadelphia: Lippincott Williams & Wilkins.

Perinchief, J. M. (2003). Documentation and management of occupational therapy services. In E. B. Crepeau, E. S. Cohn, & B. A. B. Schell (Eds.), *Willard and Spackman's occupational therapy* (10th ed., pp. 897–905). Philadelphia: Lippincott Williams & Wilkins.

Peterson, C. Q., & Nelson, D. L. (2003). Effect of an occupational intervention on printing in children with economic disadvantages. *American Journal of Occupational Therapy, 57,* 152–160.

Reed, K. L., & Sanderson, S. N. (1999). *Concepts of occupational therapy* (4th ed.). Philadelphia: Lippincott Williams & Wilkins.

Rogers, J. C., & Holm, M. B. (2003). Evaluation of areas of occupation. In E. B. Crepeau, E. S. Cohn, & B. A. B. Schell (Eds.), *Willard and Spackman's occupational therapy* (10th ed., pp. 315–363). Philadelphia: Lippincott Williams & Wilkins.

Sames, K. M. (2005). *Documenting occupational therapy practice.* Upper Saddle River, NJ: Pearson Prentice Hall.

Shumway-Cook, M., & Woollacott, M. (2001). *Motor control: Theory and practical applications.* Baltimore: Williams & Wilkins.

Soukup, M. S. (2000). The center for advanced nursing practice evidence-based practice model, evidence-based nursing practice. *Nursing Clinics of North America, 35,* 1757–1766.

Sussenberger, B. (2003). Socioeconomic factors and their influence on occupational performance. In E. B. Crepeau, E. S. Cohn, & B. A. B. Schell (Eds.), *Willard and Spackman's occupational therapy* (10th ed., pp. 97–109). Philadelphia: Lippincott Williams & Wilkins.

Taylor, R., Braveman, B., & Hammel, J. (2004). Developing and evaluating community based services through participating action research: Two case examples. *American Journal of Occupational Therapy, 58,* 73–82.

Toglia, J. P. (2005). A dynamic interactional approach to cognitive rehabilitation. In N. Katz (Ed.), *Cognition & occupation across the life span: Models for intervention in occupational therapy* (2nd ed.). Bethesda, MD: AOTA Press.

Trombly, C. A., & Ma, H. (2002). A synthesis of the effects of occupational therapy for persons with stroke, part I: Restoration of roles, tasks, and activities. *American Journal of Occupational Therapy, 56,* 250–259.

U.S. Census Bureau. (2004). American Community Survey. Retrieved June 11, 2006, from www.census.gov/hhes/www/disability/steps.html

Wilcock, A. A. (1998). *An occupational perspective of health.* Thorofare, NJ: Slack.

Wilcock, A. A. (2003). Population interventions focused on health for all. In E. B. Crepeau, E. S. Cohn, & B. A. B. Schell (Eds.), *Willard and Spackman's occupational therapy* (10th ed., pp. 30–45). Philadelphia: Lippincott Williams & Wilkins.

Wilcock, A. A. (2005). Relationship of occupations to health and well-being. In C. H. Christiansen & C. M. Baum (Eds.), *Occupational therapy performance, participation, and well-being* (3rd ed., pp. 134–165). Thorofare, NJ: Slack.

World Health Organization. (1986). A discussion document on the concept and principles of health promotion. *Health Promotion, 1,* 73–78.

World Health Organization. (2001). *International classification of functioning, disability, and health.* Geneva, Switzerland: Author.